Jessica Hatcher-Moore is a non-
awards for her reporting on wo
rights and global health issues. Born in Shropshire, she was
educated at the University of Oxford and now lives in North
Wales with her husband and two sons. *@jessiehatcher* on
Twitter and *@jessiejanehatcher* on Instagram.

Praise for *After Birth*

'An absolute treasure trove on women's physical and mental
postnatal health – information is power and information is
exactly what *After Birth* delivers'
Milli Hill, author of *Give Birth Like A Feminist* and *The
Positive Birth Book*

'Brilliant: medically wise, but also written in a very
approachable style. I think it should be prescribed reading
for all new parents'
Clover Stroud, *Sunday Times*-bestselling author of *My Wild
and Sleepless Nights*

'Important on so many levels – every new parent should
read it, men included. It is helpful, honest and humorous –
which is what we all need after birth'
Ross J. Barr, acupuncturist and women's health expert

'Essential reading for all parents-to-be'
Marina Fogle

'Such a juicy source of reliable information, delivered in
a clever and straightforward manner, with that necessary
touch of humour – this book provides an enormous public
health service to women, families and communities'
Elizabeth Braga, women's health physiotherapist

'*After Birth* provides a unique insight into the postnatal period where the focus shifts onto the baby, all too often abandoning a bewildered mum, trying to come to terms with the physical and mental aftermath of her pregnancy. It prepares you to better understand the postpartum period, be able to recognise the issues which may arise as familiar and not frightening and feel more supported and informed in the process'

Kate Walsh, pelvic-health physiotherapist and Head of Physiotherapy at Liverpool Women's Hospital

AFTER BIRTH

How to Recover Body and Mind

JESSICA HATCHER-MOORE

SOUVENIR
PRESS

This paperback edition first published in 2022

First published in Great Britain in 2021 by
Souvenir Press
an imprint of Profile Books Ltd
29 Cloth Fair
London
ECIA 7JQ

www.souvenirpress.co.uk

Illustrations: pages 35 and 253 from Artemida-psy/Shutterstock.com;
page 185 from Blamb/Shutterstock.com; pages 214, 244 and 251
by Jo Goodberry/NB Illustration

The information given within this book has been compiled to offer
general guidance on its subject and is not meant to be treated as a
substitute for qualified medical advice. Always consult a medical
practitioner before starting, stopping or changing any medical care.
Many of the women cited in this book chose not to use their
real names and so have been given pseudonyms instead.

1 3 5 7 9 10 8 6 4 2

Typeset in Berling Nova Text by MacGuru Ltd
Printed and bound in Great Britain by CPI Group (UK) Ltd, Croydon, CRO 4YY

The moral right of the author has been asserted.

A CIP catalogue record for this book is available from the British Library.

ISBN 978 1 78816 774 1
eISBN 978 1 78816 644 7

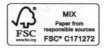

For Phil

Contents

Introduction

When my midwife estimated that our baby would weigh around seven and a half pounds, I punched the air in delight and silently praised my husband's genes. I come from a family of small, slim-hipped women who make whopper babies; seven and a half pounds was going to be a cinch. Feeling confident, I trained a laser focus on the birth. When we eventually got there, ten days late, I treated it like an athletic event that my years of cross-country and marathon running had prepared me for. The main difference was that it was now my husband, Philip, not my parents, shouting 'GO, Jess!' from the sidelines.

After 19 hours from start to finish, the baby came out and we all sank into a collapsed scrum, me clutching our precious baby to my chest and Philip somewhere beneath us. I felt ecstatic with relief: we did it, it's over. I shut my eyes, sobbing with happiness and delighting in the respite. 'Do you want to know what you've got?' the midwife asked, cutting short our reverie. I opened my eyes to see two midwives peering at us from between my thighs with curiosity.

It's a baby, I thought – a healthy baby. And then I remembered there was more to it. I obediently raised my head to see. 'It's a boy!' the midwife said, having run out of patience, and I lay back again to take in the news.

At some point after I pushed out the placenta (I'd forgotten there was an Act II), I became aware of the midwives' heads gathered again at the business end. Reality sunk in and I chastised myself for not thinking about the aftermath; labour had banished all logical thought from my mind. I'd barely had time to imagine what horrors might have befallen my vagina when the senior midwife announced there was no need for stitches – I had just a graze.

Relief once more, followed by curiosity. I knew about knees and elbows, but a grazed vagina? How? Did the baby have rough edges? Would it scab? Adrenaline coursed through my veins, keeping the pain at bay. Childbearing is glorious, I thought.

Then I put a hand down to feel my freshly grazed nether regions and almost fainted with surprise. My first thought was that there was another baby on its way, which the midwives had somehow failed to notice. My once-neat, inverted parts felt somehow bulging and elephantine. I was convinced there was a head there. Dazed, I checked that the baby was still cradled in my arms. He was – and was busy appraising me with his dark, almond-shaped eyes. So what was it? And how was I supposed to sit on it? It suddenly became clear that my physical ordeal was far from over. At the midwife's suggestion I took a bath and, as I lay back in the scarlet water, felt terrified for the first time.

*

The physical changes that result from pregnancy and childbirth encompass the wondrous, the debilitating and the downright weird. It can be like puberty all over again, with brand new bodily functions and hormones going haywire.

Women often describe this as one of the most exquisite periods in their life, with the irreplicable joy of getting to know a new human. But many also consider it one of the hardest times. For a lot of women, the shift to motherhood is the most significant mental and physical transition they're ever likely to undergo. And, in terms of your journey as a parent, it's just the prologue – the story is only beginning.

Childbirth itself can lead to a trail of physical and mental consequences that most women are unprepared for, and the gap between expectation and reality can make it hard to bear. We don't tell expectant mums that they won't necessarily love their babies immediately, that their bodies may change forever, or that up to half of them will have bladder problems even a year after the birth. We don't say there's a one in ten chance that a woman will damage the muscles of her anus during childbirth. And we don't say that as many as half of all women will experience a prolapse at some point in their lives (when the bladder, bowel or uterus drops down), likely caused by childbirth. This fallout is often described as the last taboo; most women only discover the truth when they become a medical statistic, and they often keep their problems to themselves rather than sharing them.

Instead of raising our voices about these issues, too many women accept them as the price we pay for our children, even though birth injuries are just that – injuries, which need to be fixed, and not viewed as inevitable consequences of childbirth. As a result, women are not only unprepared for problems, they are also unaware of all the therapies and treatments available that can help. Around the world, women's health is undergoing a revolution, with more and more women and men dedicating their lives to improving it. Today, no matter what the issue, there is someone who is equipped to understand, and someone who is equipped to help.

Childbirth in the UK has never been safer; stillbirth rates are decreasing and maternal mortality is becoming ever rarer. Unfortunately, however, the incidence of interventions and serious birth injuries is rising. No one knows exactly why; it's possibly because diagnostics are improving so we're recording more of these incidents, but critics blame our state maternity care, which, although it employs many dedicated individuals, is beset by budget cuts and staffing shortfalls that impact the quality of care. Eight in ten midwives say they don't have enough staff to run a safe service; their warnings must not go unheard. Critics also argue that the system can fail to recognise or pay adequate attention to what the woman goes through; a 'successful' vaginal birth, for example, includes one in which the mother is injured and unable to walk for weeks afterwards.

It's not just shortcomings in our health system but also societal factors that are to blame. We are heavier than ever – roughly 30 per cent of women in the UK are obese – which puts more strain on the muscles that support our pelvic organs and raises our chances of complications and interventions. Eating a balanced and nutritious diet while the baby is in your womb could break the cycle: it is thought to reduce the risk of your child becoming obese later in life. While this knowledge alone may not help women lose weight, it could motivate them to make better choices, or motivate others to help them to do so.

Perhaps the most significant change is that we are having children ever later. In 2000, the average age of a first-time mum was twenty-eight and a half, and by 2018 it had increased by more than two years; we are having our babies at an older age every year. The chance of complications and interventions increases with age, and the body becomes more prone to injury and less efficient at recovering. This is another reason why we need better access to the many existing channels of help.

On top of this, we are asking more of our bodies than women before us. No woman born into my grandparents' generation ever ran a marathon. (It was only in the 1970s that marathon organisers first allowed women to take part; until then, sports scientists didn't think their bodies capable of it.) And we are living longer to see minor problems worsen. A lot of expectant mums have no idea that pregnancy and delivery-related issues may only become symptomatic during or after the menopause. When problems like incontinence and prolapses do emerge, they can be treated, mostly without invasive procedures, if we can treat them in a timely manner.

Psychologists believe that the mental transition to motherhood is also getting harder. The job of mothering can feel like drudgery at times. Women with professional identities, in particular, can feel they have a lot to give up, while others struggle with the pressure to get back to work. We've also been adults for longer, so we have established our roles and routines. It seems counter-intuitive but the more proficient you are when you become a mother, the harder you may find it. In my case, life before babies tricked me into thinking that men were my equal; after the baby arrived and it was just the two of us, I felt like I understood feminism for the first time.

Lastly, we have moved away from family members who traditionally would have supported us. Wisdom that was once passed down by female relatives is not always shared. And, even if our parents are nearby, they may still be working.

Our society today champions individualism, competition and getting to the top – values that are hard to square with the first weeks and months of motherhood, when those who are able to cede control and accept imperfection are often the ones who do best. Although I can now see that making a child is the most empowering and meaningful thing I've ever done, it's taken a good couple of years for me to realise it.

*

Given the increased appetite for support during the post-natal period, you would think that care would be improving – but it's not that clear-cut. We have replaced the long hospital stays of earlier generations not with what women today want – access to physiotherapy, gynaecologists and mental health support – but with a void. The postpartum period is so neglected it's known as the Cinderella of maternity services, and this chronic lack of investment means that childbirth and recovery are not just feminist issues but political ones, too. The cuts are everywhere: there are no women's health physios on labour wards anymore, the six-week check with a doctor or nurse is rushed (if you get one at all), doctors, nurses and midwives are stretched beyond belief, and waiting lists for specialists can run into years or require you to travel hundreds of miles for treatment.

It is, however, within our power to reverse this downward trend, and you can help: by speaking out and demanding better for yourself and your children; badgering GPs and MPs and treating your pelvic floor exercises like a religion.

Before moving to North Wales, I lived in Nairobi, Kenya, where I worked as a foreign correspondent and spent most of my time on the road covering the conflicts and crises of East

Africa. I interviewed the most extraordinary women imaginable: teenagers raising the children of their rapists, women recovering from birth with no clean water let alone nappies, and mothers bringing up children in isolation, ostracised by a taboo birth injury called a fistula that had left them leaking urine for life.

I learned how devastating women's health problems can be, but also how resilient women are in the face of adversity. Not once did it occur to me that the mothers I knew back home might have faced comparable, albeit less acute, challenges. Naively, I thought leaking wee for months on end affected mothers who couldn't access healthcare, not me. I had no idea that there are women across all social strata in the UK who endure pain for years after childbirth. For some reason, I even imagined that women who stayed at home cooking, cleaning and caring for babies after their husbands departed each morning with kiss and a 'good luck' were not like me. When I married Philip, a photographer I'd met while covering the civil war in Somalia, I was a woman thriving in a man's world; I thought gender inequality didn't affect me. After we retreated to the hills of North Wales and had a baby, however, I realised how naive I'd been.

It was only after my baby emerged weighing 9lb and 5oz that my husband discovered he had weighed 9lb and 11oz at birth. At first, I was delighted; I thought I'd nailed it – a giant baby, and no stitches! Not once did it occur to me that I might be left with an embarrassing condition that my GP later described as 'normal' when I asked her for help six months later; whenever I jogged, sneezed, laughed or coughed unexpectedly, I did a mini wee.

The postnatal period is unavoidably biological, from the baby blues to the big boobs, the let-down to the inability to let go. I'd learned a lot about my mental health during my twenties and early thirties, but for some reason I struggled to apply what I knew when I needed it most as a new mother. My body with its limitations was one problem. I struggled without the endorphins and freedom I used to get from running. Claustrophobia set in. I bristled at my body's weakness; I could barely walk a mile without having to squat behind a bush. But then I also loved my body for what it had achieved. Becoming a mother is a very confusing time indeed. Resentment kicked in when Philip started leaving us every morning to renovate the cottage we'd just bought. I felt he had no idea what I was going through and, when he struggled, or just wanted some time with me alone, I resented him again for being another thing that needed me.

It was partly vanity that led me to the icy, late-autumn waters of the River Dee, which rushes below our house. I needed something to remedy the private humiliation of my physical weakness – I wanted to feel strong – so I started hurling myself into its torrent of snowmelt that runs off the mountains of Snowdonia. I swam in October, November, December, January; it was the winter of 2017, one of the coldest in years, and I swam with snow on the banks, ice underfoot and as graupel – ice-encrusted snow – fell around me. It was the perfect tonic. Every swim charged me with endorphins and adrenaline, cost nothing, took minutes (sometimes seconds) and needed no fitness, but made me feel joyously, outrageously alive, as free as the buzzard that wheeled overhead. I'm not saying all new mums should throw themselves into the nearest river to cure their postpartum woes, but we do all need to find the thing that keeps us, uniquely, sane. And then cling to it.

*

In this book, I focus on the weeks, months and – for some – years that follow birth, when you're locked into the most challenging but rewarding endurance race imaginable. Childbirth made me look at every mother with new-found respect, but in hindsight it is really just the sprint that gets you out of the starting blocks. There is no finishing line, medal or cheering crowd in this race – most of the time you're just plodding along – but the highs easily outweigh the lows, so you set your jaw and lean into the headwinds, as the extraordinary little person you have created starts to emerge.

It was a few months after my son was born that I first started asking other women about their postpartum experiences and discovered this pandemic of silent struggles, unaddressed trauma and physical hurdles that I felt was making motherhood so much harder than it needs to be. What I had experienced was just the tip of the iceberg. And I became outraged by what women around me were suffering, often without any professional support.

The legacy of one woman's birth left her in pain for years. When a doctor eventually examined her, he described her vagina as 'a bit flippy flappy' and her confidence bottomed out. Another woman went into labour convinced that it was a process her body was perfectly designed for. The expectation versus the reality – a traumatic episiotomy (a surgical cut to aid delivery) – sent her spiralling into postnatal depression. Another had an undiagnosed tear that damaged her rectum. For months, she received no guidance and had to beg her GP to examine her. What is the cost of such an experience to a new mother, I wondered? And what is the long-term cost to the State and the NHS of these problems going untreated?

Being unable to control your bladder or bowel affects two in three nursing-home residents, and is considered one of the top reasons for admission to full-time care. Our short-termist approach to postnatal rehabilitation is not only costing women their dignity, but also costing the welfare system billions of pounds.

Six months after my baby was born, I travelled to Bordeaux and discovered that the French treat pelvic floors after childbirth like the British would a disabling knee injury. Every new mother, no matter how she gave birth, sees a consultant and is sent to a specialist physiotherapist for a course of sessions that involve bespoke exercises, electric muscle stimulation and biofeedback to ensure the complete 're-education' of her pelvic floor, while another specialist rehabilitates her abdominal muscles. When I learned about the French approach, I felt staggered by the disservice we do women in the UK.

Attitudes here are changing and the taboo is fading. More women actually know what they look like down below, for a start. But there are fresh challenges. We see airbrushed images of postpartum celebrities showing off washboard stomachs weeks after giving birth. More women than ever are requesting cosmetic surgery on their vulvas. And, because postnatal healthcare is neglected, women are bypassing their doctors to seek solutions on their own, becoming vulnerable to well-meaning but misinformed peers, celebrities and quacks. I had one rule in pregnancy: never google symptoms, because I invariably just search for the answer I want. I mostly stuck to it, but when the baby arrived I was online again, anxiously searching 'haemorrhoids' or 'prolapse' because personal experience dictated that I would not get what I needed from my GP.

The postpartum period is defined by changes – to your body, your life, your relationships and your coping strategies. To keep up with these, you do need information. But you need good information. This book provides that. It is unbiased (I have no stake in the healthcare industry), evidence-based, and includes the opinions of hundreds of experts from diverse disciplines. It is also – I hope – a friend to whom you can turn when you're feeling unsure. I share my own stories and those of other mothers to remind you that you're not alone. These women tell their stories with characteristic guts and humour, and it was their strength and honesty that initially fired up the reporter in me. Among them are some of the most impressive women I know – human rights lawyers, doctors, and the founders and CEOs of businesses. If they aren't getting the help they badly need, how are postpartum struggles affecting the most vulnerable and marginalised in our society? As with so many women's health issues, there is almost no research on the subject.

One of the most common criticisms I encountered of the book's premise was: 'Won't it put women off having children?' I don't think so. Having children may be one of the hardest things you'll ever do, but no woman that I've met questions whether it was worth it. They would just like to have been better prepared. As one pelvic health physiotherapist told me, you never meet a woman who is cross at having been over-prepared for this beautiful and formative time in her and her baby's life, only under-prepared. 'Confidence is knowing the truth,' she said.

Before a knee operation, consultants detail all the risks and describe the recovery process so that patients can make informed decisions and, if something goes wrong, be braced for it. Why is it so different for childbirth? In a recent UK study, midwives told expectant mums at 36 weeks all about the risks of vaginal childbirth, including the rates of serious tears that damaged the anus, versus the risks of a caesarean. Many expected it to cause the caesarean rate to rise – but it stayed the same. The hypno-birthing mantras that celebrate our bodies' ability to give life through this natural process are not at odds with the fact that, more often than not, childbirth is somehow medicalised – and it's condescending to assume women can't comprehend that duality. The 37 trillion cells that make up a woman's body are arranged with awe-inspiring perfection, but this doesn't make our bodies invulnerable to injury.

I want women in future generations to talk and read as much, if not more, about the postpartum period as they do about pregnancy and birth. Whatever your birth is like, you will need a lot of support afterwards – particularly if you have twins or more. Surround yourself with people to help you, and information you trust. You don't need to read this book cover to cover; read the parts that apply to you now, then save the rest for reference later.

In part one, the first chapter describes the phenomenal feats of human reproduction. The following two chapters are written for women who want to know what they can do before birth to prepare. Part two is arranged by body part and deals with the first six weeks postpartum, and part three, again arranged by body part, covers the longer-term effects of pregnancy, childbirth and motherhood. The final section is written for partners, to help them understand what women go through postnatally, to better understand what they themselves might be going through, and to put them in a stronger position to help.

You may not – and I hope you don't – encounter any of

the problems I discuss in the book, but if you do, I hope the information included here helps you to spend more time enjoying yourself and less time worrying as you ride the highs and lows of pregnancy and motherhood. It is the book I'd give to my sister and to my daughter, and the book I wish my mother had given to me. I hope it will empower women of all ages to know themselves better and to seek the best for their minds and bodies. And it comes with a personal guarantee: if something peculiar, uncomfortable or traumatic is going on with you, then there's another woman, somewhere, experiencing the same thing.

1

The Making of a Mum

I'm starting here with a canter through what happens to your body when you conceive and grow a baby, because it's difficult to care about and engage with something – in this case, your body – if you don't understand it. The bombardment of physical and mental challenges during pregnancy, childbirth and early motherhood are without comparison – other than, perhaps, the transition through puberty. For too long, however, the story of childbirth has begun with a fantasy, in which a woman's egg is prey to the heroic sperm, which journeys through a maelstrom of challenges to beat off opponents and arrive victorious at the ovum; this egg, meanwhile, waits like a princess in her ivory tower for natural selection to ensure the fastest and fittest candidate arrives. In reality, there is rather more nuance to it than that. But, while our laws and customs have changed to give women as much agency as men in daily life, the fairy tale of valorous sperm cells doing all the work is proving harder to shift.

Sperm are more accurately portrayed as stumbling drunkards with no sense of direction, and the woman's body is anything but passive. It is only the dynamic crowd-control measures employed by the cervix, a cylinder of dense tissue that separates the vagina from the womb, that manages to cajole the sperm into useful service; the cervix keeps the sperm in holding pens and releases them in stages to flow up towards the egg. One of the few things sperm seem good at is surviving; they have been found in the little caves that the cervix creates for them for as long as nine days after ejaculation. It's unclear how exactly the sperm make it to the egg – whether by chance or because the cervix and uterus, with its channels of thinned-out mucus, draw them in – but, if one does manage to pass through the egg's outer layer, she immediately initiates a lockdown procedure to protect herself from further sperm who might attempt to join the party. And with that, the making of a human being, and a mother, begins.

By the time your due date comes around, you may be rueing the day your body guided in that sperm. You are likely more than two stone heavier, and every one of the major systems in your body – heart, lungs, blood, liver, kidneys and digestive system – has changed dramatically to cope with the demands of the fetus. In terms of energy expenditure, you are running at twice your normal metabolic rate, close to the upper limit of what the human body can endure. Some scientists believe that hitting this point, which is known as our metabolic ceiling, is what dictates when the baby needs to come out.

One day, around 38 weeks after conception, a miracle happens. Something – scientists don't know exactly what – calls time on the fetus' repose and kickstarts a dazzlingly complex cascade of events that eject it into the world. Firstly, your body starts making enormous quantities of prostaglandins, which it usually produces in response to pain or illness. In this case, the hormones stimulate uterine contractions, which push the baby down into the birth canal. If you need help getting to this point, doctors apply prostaglandins in the form of a gel to get things going. This is called induction.

Assuming all goes well and the cervix – the baby's gateway into the world – has opened in the process we know as dilation, the baby's head now needs to navigate the narrow birth canal that tunnels through the bones and musculature of the pelvis and includes the cervix, vagina and external vulva. This is the tricky part. At its narrowest point, the birth canal is often smaller than the baby's head, a problem that has been at the heart of human evolutionary theory for over half a century. In order to give birth to big-brained babies, we need wide pelvises, but it's narrow pelvises that are best for running and walking. This apparent conundrum is known as the obstetrical dilemma. If the theory holds true, it means that our species' progress has imposed on us a risky trade-off: we give birth only fractionally before our baby's head grows too big. Animals, by comparison, tend to give birth much later in their infants' development process; lambs totter around and nibble grass when they're just days old.

Whatever it is that limits human gestation, we don't always get the timing right, which is why the second stage of labour can be so hard – but also why evolution has given us a playbook of tricks. Our babies' heads and brains have the ability to change shape quite dramatically as they are squeezed out, forming a cone to help them through the narrow aperture. The bones and ligaments in our normally rigid pelvises also flex. And women with large heads, who are likely to have babies with large heads, tend to have pelvises that can accommodate their large-headed progeny.

When the baby is ready to descend through the birth canal, your contours and contractions cause it to tuck in its chin, then the pelvic floor muscles channel it into a series of complex rotations. If the baby completes these, it will successfully navigate the irregularly shaped pelvis so that its head, followed by shoulders and body, exit the vagina. And with that, mother (in the literal sense) and baby are born.

While this may sound manageable, it is rare that a woman – and particularly a first-timer – delivers her baby then remarks upon the immaculate design of Mother Nature. Childbirth is a staggering, empowering and sometimes devastating trial, where any deviation from the norm – if the baby has its hand up by its face, or if one or another phase of labour is too long or not long enough – could result in injury to the mother, baby or both.

Hot on the baby's heels comes the placenta, which until this point has been the baby's engine room, producing phenomenal quantities of oestrogen and progesterone – more than your body will make in total during the rest of your life – that maintained the optimal environment for your baby's development. When the placenta leaves your body, your hormone levels start to drop. This initiates another complicated chain of events that flips the switch on your milk factories.

Your breasts have already been enlarged by the milk-making ducts that you've produced during pregnancy. Each has increased its volume by around 100ml and transformed into a powerful production plant full of tiny tubes (ducts) and sacs (alveoli) that transport and store your milk. The skin covering them will look thinner than usual, and the blood vessels will be more prominent; this is because the blood flow to your breasts has by now doubled. The nipples are also larger and more erect and the areolas more pigmented than before; it is thought that this is to attract the newborn baby like beacons. Babies are born with the urge to get to their mother's nipple; placed on a mother's abdomen and left to its own devices, almost every newborn will crawl up until it finds a nipple and start suckling within an hour, a phenomenon first described by Swedish academics in the late eighties.

Initially, your breasts produce colostrum, that fabled liquid gold so rich in wonder products such as antioxidants, antibodies and other immune cells that it is considered a new frontier in medical science; colostrum from cows is already being used to fight infections, repair tissue, boost athletic performance and improve gut health. In these first hours and days after birth, your body interprets early and regular suckling on your nipples as a cue to set up your milk supply proper. After a few days, your breasts will swell inordinately with your first batch of milk and, within a week or two, your mature milk – a substance just as miraculous as colostrum – will be established. As long as your infant suckles regularly, your body should continue to produce milk.

Whenever the baby suckles, your body produces oxytocin, the hormone you produce when you fall in love, cuddle or orgasm. It tells the muscles surrounding the sacs to contract, pushing milk into the nine or so openings of your nipple. This process is known as the 'let-down', and anything from a curious tingling sensation to full-on agony can accompany it. Your body quickly establishes a positive feedback loop, so that the more your baby suckles, the more milk you make.

Breastmilk includes over 200 different components and, in terms of composition, changes constantly – from colostrum to mature milk, fore milk (which you produce at the start of a feed) to hind milk (which you produce towards the end), from morning milk to evening milk (which is higher in sleep-inducing substances), and from milk for newborns to milk for toddlers. The number of antibodies in breastmilk also varies. Some scientists even believe that your nipples take in minute quantities of infant backwash, which your body then analyses. If their saliva shows signs of infection, or so the theory goes, then your body loads your breast milk with extra antibodies to fight it; this could explain how and why the antibody composition of breastmilk is forever changing.

Levels of relaxin, the hormone that softens your ligaments and connective tissues to allow the baby out, drop sharply after birth but are still much higher than normal if you're breastfeeding. This is why women are told to take extra care with their bodies during and after pregnancy – their joints are less stable. Scientists aren't sure why levels of relaxin remain high during breastfeeding, but relaxin is present in breastmilk and it's possible that it is one of the many substances that help the newborn's stomach and gut to develop.

The fact that the baby is still so dependent on its mother after birth has led to the phrase 'the fourth trimester'. Recalling the obstetrical dilemma, it's because our babies have such big brains but we need such small pelvises that they are born far earlier than evolution would like. A typical baby doubles in size during the first six months and, if you are breastfeeding exclusively, this will be one of the most metabolically challenging events in your life. At one month old, the typical infant needs 500 calories per day, and by six months old, this will have risen to around 650 calories each day – all from you.

Although demanding, breastfeeding is extremely good for a woman's body. It leaves you with an improved metabolism long after you've stopped feeding, so that you're better at metabolising fats and sugars than you were before. Scientists don't know for sure, but it's possible this explains the link between breastfeeding and lower rates of breast cancer, ovarian cancer, diabetes and obesity later in life.

Around the same time that your milk comes in, your levels of oestrogen and progesterone are lower than ever. These key hormones govern your menstrual cycle, but also regulate the levels of happy hormones, serotonin and dopamine in your brain. It takes a while for your body to replenish its stocks and, until then, you're vulnerable to anxiety and depression. This is why so many women – almost 80 per cent by some estimates – experience the 'baby blues', when they want to cry inexplicably and feel anxious and depressed for a short period after the birth.

The moment your baby is born, your body begins the natural process of returning to something like its pre-pregnancy state. Your cervix, which previously looked like a tightly closed sea anemone, took a battering during the birth and now hangs down, limp and long, leaving the road to your uterus wide open. Your uterus is empty now but still weighs roughly a kilo, over 16 times its normal weight, and fills half of your tummy. Your vulva, vagina and perineum – the multiple layers of muscle between the vagina and back passage – may be damaged if you had a vaginal birth; cuts or tears through the tissue may need stitching. The nerves that connect your pelvic area to your brain can also be stretched or compressed, meaning your body's signals – such as when you need to go to the loo – aren't working properly.

The pelvic floor is the scaffolding that holds up your organs. A muscular sling, it connects to your pelvis at the front and back and has three gaps in it – one for your anus, one for your urethra and one for your vagina. By the time you went into labour, the muscles, connective tissue and liga-ments of the pelvic floor were already weakened by the sheer weight of your pregnant state and softened by relaxin. During birth itself, the muscles can stretch by up to three times their normal length, become compressed, or tear. It's believed that around 20 per cent of women emerge from their first vaginal birth with pelvic floor muscles that have partially detached from the bony structure of the pelvis – an injury that may be asymptomatic, at least for now.

When you breastfeed, oxytocin also tells your uterus to start shrinking back into the pelvis, so that your bladder, bowel and pelvic organs can return to their original place. It takes around ten days to heal the plate-sized wound in your uterus where the placenta was once attached, and roughly six weeks for the cervix and uterus to go back into place. You'll be bleeding for three to four weeks as your body cleans out the uterus; the lochia, as this bleeding is known, becomes progressively lighter in colour as you heal, until it becomes colourless. If you had a caesarean, you have an additional wound that needs to heal, where the surgeon had to cut through half a dozen layers of tissue to reach your baby. The body needs a rich mix of nutrients to repair all of the damaged tissue, so a varied diet at this stage is vital.

Around the world, women practise a traditional period of rest, or 'lying-in', that coincides with the lochia; for 30 to 40 days, new mothers rest at home with their newborns while breastfeeding and being cared for by others. In most Western cultures, the medical establishment considers six weeks to be the cut-off point for postpartum recovery. When asked, however, women say on average that it takes a year to feel recovered, and up to two years for the abdominal muscles to regain their tone. How long it will take you depends on a number of factors, including your genetics, what sort of labour you had, and how long you breastfeed for – if at all.

While you are now, in the technical sense, a mother, anthropologists and psychologists believe you are only just beginning your metamorphosis. The term they use to describe the transition to motherhood is matrescence. The *Cambridge English Dictionary* defines it as the process of becoming a mother, encompassing the 'physical, psychological and emotional changes you go through after the birth of your child', noting that these have been largely unexplored by the medical community. Matrescence is marked by distinct chemical alterations in your brain that lead to mood changes, psychological obstacles, and a huge identity shift. Becoming a mother is, as the American psychologist Alexandra Sacks writes, 'one of the most significant physical and psychological changes a woman will ever experience', and it can be just as demanding as childbirth.

We don't fully understand these changes, but puberty – something we know more about – provides helpful clues. During puberty, surges of oestrogen and progesterone similar to those seen during pregnancy cause the teenage brain to undergo a remodelling process, in preparation for adulthood. Unused neural connections leftover from childhood are cut back and the brain is sculpted into its mature form. These hormonal and neurological changes are linked to what we all know – that teenagers can be moody, unpredictable and emotionally vulnerable. What most people don't realise is that pregnant women go through a very similar thing: their brains are pruned and sculpted again into a new form that is optimised to care for a baby, as described by scientists at the Universitat Autònoma de Barcelona in 2016.

A new mother's brain is, physically, smaller than it was before, but less can be more when it comes to brain matter. Pregnancy pruning only happens in the regions associated with emotional attachment and empathy. It's possible that it sacrifices certain areas of memory in favour of other things

– which might explain why you forget your friend's name or why you walked into a shop. Some even believe that the pruning may help the mother to forget the pain of childbirth. Overall, however, your ability to learn, reason and understand remains unchanged, but your ability to empathise is enhanced.

Brain-pruning focuses a mother's mind on her baby, so that she becomes more attuned to its needs. Neuroscientists can actually predict how attached a mother is to her baby just by looking at how much grey matter she has lost – if significant pruning has taken place, she is likely very well attached.

The hormone oxytocin is also busy improving your bond with your baby – as it does throughout the animal kingdom. It increases vigilance, improves your ability to read facial expressions and cues, and provides those mushy feelings that hold you hostage to your baby. It even makes your baby's head smell good; the smell of a two-day-old baby has the same giddy effect on a woman's brain as an unexpected present or recreational drug, even if she's not the child's mother and has never given birth, which is why scientists liken motherhood to falling in love.

What we don't know is how exactly these adaptations map onto behavioural changes, and how our experiences feed into them. What's clear, however, is that 'mummy brain', 'baby brain' or 'mumnesia' is not about deficiencies but is in fact a complex interplay of biology, experiences, relationships and memories.

Dr Alexandra Sacks puts the psychological changes of motherhood broadly into four categories: family dynamics – because you have not just created a baby, you've created a family; ambivalence – the contradictions of wanting your child close whilst craving space, or loving and hating parenting, sometimes at the same time; the gap between your expectations and reality; and new feelings of guilt, shame and failure that often arise.

Having navigated all of this, the woman becomes a mother – and, in many cases, nature and culture contrive one last miracle: the urge to do it again!

Part 1

PREHAB – PREPARING FOR BIRTH

At some point during the third trimester, my midwife told me that horse-riders are reputed to have iron-like perineums that refuse to give way to crowning infants. Dismayed, I told her I'd been riding horses since before I could walk. Weeks later I read that, contrary to what I believed, doing pelvic floor exercises during pregnancy could actually prolong labour if the muscles were tight. Being naturally muscly, and mistakenly equating a rigid perineum with a strong pelvic floor, I thought that if anyone had an unyielding pelvic floor, surely it would be me. Embracing the proverb 'if in doubt, do nowt', I stopped doing pelvic floor exercises altogether. Sadly, this proved to be the wrong call – my pelvic floor muscles turned out not to be that strong or responsive, and I suffered as a result.

This section contains the many things I wish I'd known about my body before giving birth. The information in these pages could reduce your chances of sustaining a birth injury, prepare you for the challenging period of recovery, and start to bridge the gap between expectation and reality that so often floors new mums. All the women I've spoken to for this book agree on one thing: that our culture neglects women's physical and mental needs during the postnatal period and fails to prepare them for it. There are myriad external factors behind this, from budget cuts to the values society prizes in women nowadays. But there are also personal factors at play.

In my case, pregnancy forced on me a degree of disconnect from my body; it looked so unfamiliar, and started doing such unpredictable things, that it was not really mine anymore. I had no control over it, and that alarmed me. Whether I would end up with belly folds like the underside of a field mushroom was out of my hands, so I started to ignore it, and applied the same fatalism to the postnatal period. What kind of birth I'd have, what kind of baby I'd get, whether I'd get postnatal depression, whether I'd have to sit on a doughnut-shaped cushion for three months, or whether I'd bounce straight back – I had no control over any of this, so I decided there was no point in preparing.

What I didn't realise was that birth is an ordeal for every woman and that, no matter what yours is like, you should prepare for a significant period of rest and recovery afterwards. In the West, many mums say that it takes a year or more to feel themselves again. Perhaps if we were more careful with ourselves during the first month or so, we would recover more swiftly in the long run.

It's important to know that you can influence many aspects of your recovery – particularly those that relate to nutrition, sleep and physical rehabilitation. Instead of disconnecting from your body in the final stages of pregnancy, as I did, experts recommend that you engage closely with it – in particular your most intimate parts, because they will soon need your full attention. As Maisie Hill writes in the book *Period Power*, 'A simple act of revolution is to learn about your body.'

2

During Pregnancy

If you're planning a vaginal birth, someone should tell you that the contours of your vagina (the internal part) and vulva (the external part) may change; if you can get to know them before the birth, it'll help when it comes to your recovery. Someone should also tell you that more than 85 per cent of women delivering vaginally will have some sort of tear or an episiotomy, according to the NCT, and that at least a third of women will require stitches. Having stitches isn't usually the nightmare scenario that childless women envisage, but a routine procedure. And not having stitches is not necessarily the holy grail, either; I didn't have any stitches, despite my outsize child, but I had more problems getting back into exercise than some women who tore through multiple layers of tissue did.

It's very natural, when you're approaching labour, to put your fingers in your ears when you hear all of this stuff and say, 'I'm just going to go to hospital and do whatever they tell me, because they know best.' But this is your body, and no one else cares about it like you do. Childbirth can have a huge impact on it, so don't sign over all the decisions to a group of strangers. Engage with your body, particularly now, before you give birth, so that you are invested in the decisions you'll need to make during labour, and so that you'll know what you need to feel supported, before, during and afterwards.

Know your pelvic floor

The pelvic floor is like a hammock of muscles and tissue strung between your coccyx (or tailbone) at the back and your pubic bone at the front. It's impossible to overstate how important these muscles are to your body, now and in the future. They are the bedrock of your abdomen, supporting your bladder, bowel and uterus, and will get progressively weaker as you age. Somewhere between 10 and 20 per cent of us will one day undergo surgery for a prolapse – when one of the three pelvic organs drops down because the pelvic floor muscles aren't supporting it. This condition is thought to affect up to 50 per cent of women during their lifetime (although some will be asymptomatic) and the number one cause is pregnancy. About a third of women will also suffer urinary incontinence, and somewhere between 5 and 25 per cent struggle to control bowel movements or gas. If you can make sure that your muscles are strong and supple before going into labour, you can improve your chances of an intervention-free labour, prevent incontinence after birth and reduce your chances of incontinence or a prolapse later in life.

Train the muscles before birth

In 2004, Kjell Å Salvesen and Siv Mørkved, two Norwegian experts in pelvic health, found that doing structured pelvic floor muscle training between weeks 20 and 36 of pregnancy lowered the chances of actively pushing in labour for more than 60 minutes – and it's this active pushing stage that is the most risky for your baby and can cause the most damage to your body. This isn't because you need strong pelvic floor muscles for labour (they need to be relaxed for the baby

29

to come out), but, physiotherapists say, because you need to know how to relax them when you're pushing. A 2017 Cochrane Review, the gold standard for medical evidence and decision-making, showed that supervised pelvic floor muscle training during pregnancy also reduced symptoms of incontinence in late pregnancy and after birth. If you train the muscles now, you'll have better residual strength and a better understanding of how to strengthen them afterwards. As physios have told me, it can be very hard to get them functioning well again after birth if you had no connection to them before.

Make sure you can feel them lift and then lower

Before you start pelvic floor muscle training, it's important to know whether your muscles can tense and release normally. Can you contract the same muscles that stop a wee, or hold a fart? Can you feel them lift as you tense, and lower as you release, without moving your buttocks at all? When you put a finger inside your vagina and tense, can you feel a squeeze? And then a release? If so, you probably have a functional pelvic floor (in which case, see Chapter 15 for more on pelvic floor strength training).

If you can't feel the muscles drop down or release when you relax, it may be that they have become short and tense – too tense to release, in fact. This can happen for a number of reasons, including physical or mental trauma, tension and stress, or holding on to the muscles without releasing for too long, for example, at the gym or if you have any signs of incontinence. An overactive pelvic floor is also linked to painful sex, constipation and pelvic pain, amongst other things, so if this sounds like you, see a pelvic health physiotherapist, as you may need to down-train your pelvic floor in order to ensure the muscles can relax during birth.

Meet the vagina whisperers

Women's health physios – who I refer to as pelvic health physios, because many also work with men – are like detectives who hunt for the root cause of a problem by gathering disparate clues. Their enthusiasm for all things related to the pelvis is contagious; they consider the pelvic floor to be the most underrated organ in the body. But it doesn't stop there – their work incorporates psychology, spinal health, posture, gait and any number of other factors that have a bearing on the pelvic area.

If you haven't come across them before, you will after childbirth. Around the world, this (largely female) army of vagina whisperers wants to bring about a revolution in how we talk about and care for our private parts. The NHS-sponsored app, Squeezy, now has a directory that lists all pelvic health physios in the UK and provides details of how to access them – privately, via the NHS, or both – and whether you can refer yourself or need a doctor to do so.

These physios would love for all pregnant women to see a pelvic health physio in their second trimester. Pelvic floor dysfunction is becoming more common – particularly too-tight pelvic floors – and as many as 80 per cent of women do pelvic floor exercises wrong. If anything doesn't feel right, see your GP and ask for a referral, or refer yourself; the protocol is different in each NHS Trust, but lots of physios, particularly in England, accept referrals. If that doesn't work, or you have no symptoms but want to safeguard your future health and continence, private care is widespread. At upwards of £50 for an initial session, it's expensive, but a 2019 study found that parents in the UK spend on average £10,000 on baby gear and preparations in the first year of their child's life (including £1,500 on childcare, £650 on buggies and a staggering £1,000 on clothes) – and 90 per cent admit afterwards that they wasted money. Investing in your long-term health at this point will never be a waste of money, and it may well be the smartest investment you ever make for your child. Consider it an insurance policy for your joint wellbeing, because they're going to need you in good shape for a while.

Don't ignore your BMI

When I was first pregnant, a friend gave me the bestselling book *The Best Friends' Guide To Pregnancy*. By page one I wanted to throw it in the bin. The book's author is scathing of women who gain no more than the recommended amount of weight, and of women who 'actually ask questions at the childbirth preparedness classes'. Instead, women should surrender and 'EAT', based on the fact that society is suspicious of skinny pregnant women, and that no one ever called a pregnant woman fat. The author is also strongly opposed to exercise during pregnancy because, amongst other reasons, you won't look good in Lycra, and exercise 'will not help you in Labor or Delivery in Any Way'.

It's hard to justify any of this advice. Research shows that your weight during pregnancy, childbirth and postpartum does matter – for your health and that of the baby – and the more you gain during pregnancy (and the more overweight you were before becoming pregnant), the harder it'll be to lose it afterwards. Your Body Mass Index (or BMI) is an imperfect but commonly used measure of body fat that's based on weight and height. In the UK, the average 25- to 34-year-old woman's BMI is 26.9, which is classed as 'overweight'. This already puts a majority of women into a higher-risk category for pregnancy, childbirth and beyond. Most women simply don't have much of a margin to 'pack on the pounds' without potentially making things harder for themselves or their babies.

Weight also factors into pelvic floor problems like prolapses, because being heavier puts more pressure on your pelvic floor. Researchers recently discovered that around 20 per cent of women who have a vaginal birth end up with an injury to their pelvic floor known as an avulsion, where the deep muscle partially detaches from their pubic bone. If you imagine the main muscle in your pelvic floor as a tent, with guy ropes and pegs pulling it taut at the front and the back, an avulsion means one or both of the guy ropes at the front are severed, so your tent will never be quite as solid again. Avulsion is considered the leading cause of prolapses – and one of the only things that is shown to prevent it is to control your BMI during pregnancy.

You don't need to eat for two

The cliché that you're eating for two during pregnancy has now been debunked – you don't need a great deal more food than normal to build a baby, but you do need a diet that's high in nutrients. (For more on this, see Chapter 9, because the diet that is recommended postpartum is pretty much the same as during pregnancy.) Your extra calorie intake needs to build up to between 200 and 300 calories per day by the third trimester; nutritionist Lily Nichols says it's more like eating for 1.1 people, rather than two.

You can – and should – exercise

If you have a normal, healthy pregnancy and it is safe for you to do so, know that exercising during pregnancy is linked to a healthy mother and child. A growing body of evidence shows that moderate exercise is associated with a reduced risk of conditions such as pre-eclampsia (a complication characterised by high blood pressure), hypertension, diabetes, miscarriage and pre-term labour, and that the benefits to the baby persist into childhood, with healthy growth and even, according to some, higher cognitive abilities and intelligence. 'Overall, the benefits of exercise during pregnancy decrease the risk of chronic disease for both mother and child', a 2016 review of scientific literature concludes.

Listen to your body

Somewhere in between these evidence-based recommendations and the outdated notion that you should eat for two lies your personal trajectory, which will be informed by your own reality. In my case, nausea during the first trimester led me to subsist on breakfast cereal, biscuits and toast, and I felt so exhausted I barely left the sofa. And then, in the second and third trimesters, I suddenly felt like indulging in red meat, berries, nuts and seeds, full-fat yoghurt, cheese, avocados, eggs, milk, as well as dark chocolate and cake, taking long walks and, if I felt like it, jogging gently. Once you're through the first trimester of wanting to subsist on crisps and Pot Noodles (don't worry too much – it's a phase), if you can tune in to what your body wants and mostly eat foods that are high in nutrients, proteins and healthy fats rather than empty carbs like white bread, you'll be helping yourself and your baby through labour and beyond.

THE VULVA

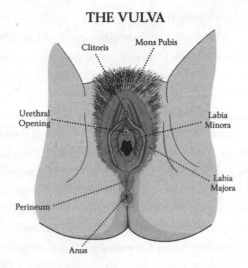

Clitoris

Mons Pubis

Urethral
Opening

Labia
Minora

Labia
Majora

Perineum

Anus

Massage your perineum

It's not just an excuse for a kinky massage; research shows that massaging the muscle tissue of your perineum – or, more literally, stretching it – prior to birth increases your chances of keeping it intact. The NHS says it is particularly helpful with your first birth, or if you have scar tissue or a rigid perineum. It's also the ideal opportunity to acquaint yourself with an area that is likely to require some attention after you give birth. From 34 weeks onwards, every day or every other day, the NHS recommends you use a couple of drops of unscented, organic oil as lubrication and place clean thumbs just inside your vagina at the back where it meets the perineum. There's no way, at 37 weeks pregnant, that I could have got both my thumbs down there at once, so you might want to settle for one – or get your partner to help, in which case they'll probably use their index fingers, not thumbs. Pressing down towards your bottom and the sides, run your thumb(s) around the opening at the back wall of the vagina in a U-shaped manoeuvre so that you feel it stretching. You can also push down and to the sides until you feel a bit of burning and hold that stretch for a minute or two. Relax as much as you can while you do this, and aim for around five minutes each time.

> *Clare Bourne, a pelvic health physiotherapist in London, on women's reluctance to massage their perineums:*
> 'Sometimes I speak to women and they say, "that's disgusting". This is often our overall attitude to the vagina – that it's a bit weird, and that you shouldn't touch it too much. So how about getting your husband to do it? "Oh no," they say. "I wouldn't want my husband to do that." Then we're back to children and birth being a woman's thing; something men don't get involved in. We're trying to get through to women without scaremongering. Hearing what can happen during labour is scary, but it's far more scary when you're out the other side having had no preparation for it. Being ignorant is less scary initially, but we don't consider the impact of that choice. After giving birth, none of my clients ever come back to my clinic angry that they were over-informed – women are only ever angry that they were under-informed.'

Are serious injuries an inevitable consequence of childbirth?

No. It's wrongly assumedly by some in the medical profession that third- and fourth-degree tears – known in the trade as Obstetric Anal Sphincter Injuries, or OASIs (see page 64) – from your vagina into your back passage are an inevitable consequence of vaginal birth. These injuries can lead to problems with bowel and bladder control, amongst other things, and have a significant impact psychologically.

In Finland, OASI rates (which have been stable for the last 25 years) are less than 1 per cent, while in the UK they have tripled since 2000 to around 6 per cent; if you're over 35, your risk is higher. The reason these serious injuries are so rare in Finland is thought to be down to their policy of manually supporting the perineum during all vaginal births – known as 'the Finnish grip' or 'hands-on' childbirth (see page 45). Rather than accept the UK's current rate of birth injuries as inevitable, we should be calling for more investment in maternal and postnatal care. The future of childbirth lies in better information. At the University of Michigan, doctors have been modelling the effects of labour on a woman's body. Their results suggest that around 75 per cent of women should be able to give birth to a baby of any size without injury, while roughly 10 per cent of women risk injury delivering a baby of any head size. Ultimately, their goal is for a woman to have an assessment of her birth canal relative to the size of the baby's head before going into labour, so she can make an informed choice about how to give birth and avoid injury. This sort of approach is the future, but we're going to need to raise our voices in order to see it.

Be informed

Giving birth in the UK is safer now than at any point in our history. Despite the movement that has encouraged women to have 'natural' births, however, the number of medical interventions during birth is increasing in the UK. In legal terms, a woman's autonomy is paramount when it comes to childbirth, meaning you must be the primary decision-maker, not your midwife or doctor; it is illegal to do anything to you without your consent. A growing body of evidence shows that, no matter what interventions your birth might involve, you are likely to have a positive experience if you are well informed of what might happen and feel in control of the decisions you make.

The question is, how do you inform yourself without frightening yourself? The Royal College of Obstetricians and Gynaecologists produces a series of patient information leaflets (see Resources) written for pregnant women planning their birth, and many NHS Trusts have their own leaflets. These should, however, be a starting point, says Birth Rights, the UK charity for protecting women's rights in childbirth, because everyone's situation is different. A 42-year-old having her first baby conceived by IVF, for example, has very different concerns to a 22-year-old wanting a large family.

Many women complain after birth that they felt patronised or infantilised by medical staff during labour. Milli Hill, the author of *Give Birth Like a Feminist*, urges perinatal women to behave 'in the same strong, grown-up way that you behave in other areas of your life, such as your career or your relationship.' Don't be afraid to ask for evidence, and for the risks and benefits to be clearly explained.

A conversation should happen with your midwife or doctor during early pregnancy. This will be about normal pregnancy and normal delivery. It should include the risk factors for birthing problems that might affect you, together with reassurance about how often or not such issues and injuries occur, what can prevent them and what can repair them. As pregnancy progresses, if at any point it becomes clear that there is the possibility of needing a caesarean section, then the pros and cons of this will be discussed.

In the same way, if you are allowed to go into labour, the expectation is that you will have a normal delivery. In some cases, due to risk factors, the chance of an intervention being required during a vaginal birth is considered greater, in which case the pros and cons of that intervention will be discussed. As situations evolve during labour, further counselling will take place.

Healthcare providers are legally obliged to have a personalised conversation with you about the risks and benefits of any action, taking into account your situation and what is important to you. This may be a challenge, especially where immediate action is necessary to safeguard you and your baby, but ideally it is what we women need to maintain dignity and respect in childbirth.

A lot of women I interviewed criticised organisations like the NCT for their blinkered focus on 'natural' birth when, more often than not, some external intervention is involved. We can get very het up about instrumental deliveries here in the UK, but when I spoke to a friend in France hours after she gave birth with the help of a ventouse cap, it reminded me that interventions needn't be a negative thing at all. 'It was great, my partner was amazing, and I had a ventouse because I'd been pushing for two hours – but they didn't need to cut me and I didn't have any tears.' The best obstetricians, both here in the UK and elsewhere, have the skills to deliver babies safely *and* minimise damage to the women in all but extreme cases.

Today, good medical practice typically involves patients and doctors making decisions together, in partnership, with each listening to the others' views and the doctor providing all the information the patient needs to make an informed choice. With financial constraints and staffing shortages, however, and maternity services being asked to do more with less, this isn't always possible; there's only usually one consultant on a labour ward, so they may not be available to answer questions; it is hoped that other qualified staff will be.

Ultimately, as an obstetrician reminds me, what matters above all to your medical team is that they deliver a healthy baby in good condition – which is, one can only assume, in line with what you want, too. But don't equate that with thinking that your experience of birth doesn't matter; it matters a great deal.

Remember three questions…

The Royal College of Obstetricians and Gynaecologists suggests you start by getting answers to the following three questions if you are asked to make a choice about your healthcare. It's too much to start thinking about them for the first time during labour, so explore them beforehand:

1. What are my options?
2. What are the pros and cons of each option for me?
3. How do I get support to help me make a decision that is right for me?

Jemima's health team ignored her request for a caesarean and, rather than asking for consent, told her she was to be induced. She got her caesarean, but only when the induction failed, she was septic, and her baby was in distress:
'I'd spoken to lots of people who'd had bad birth experiences. I didn't want a birth at home with jungle song but I did feel strongly that we're either doing this naturally or I want a C-section; I didn't want anything in between. At

*NCT classes, you are wholly focused on giving birth natu-
rally. Where is the practical discussion about other things?
There were ten of us in my class, and five of us ended up
having emergency C-sections, all because we'd had a premature rupture of the membrane. Why didn't they prepare us
for that? Women nowadays are so much more clued up, why
wouldn't we talk about it? The main thing I say to my friends
now is, inform yourself, so that you're not suddenly in a situation where you don't have control. I didn't give consent for
anything they did to me. As a nurse, I'm realising more and
more that my patients know themselves the best, and if they
tell me something, I will act on it.'*

Elective caesareans

It's within your rights to choose how you give birth, and that
choice includes requesting a caesarean. NICE, the UK's pre-
mier health watchdog, says that NHS Trusts should always
offer planned caesareans to women who, after discussion
and support, say that a vaginal birth is still not an acceptable
option. In reality, however, only 26 per cent of trusts offer
caesareans in line with these best-practice guidelines, almost
half of all trusts had problematic or inconsistent policies and
practices, and 15 per cent actively do not support caesareans
requested by mothers.

Prepare for the postpartum period

It's common – and telling – that women often regret putting
all their effort into preparation for the birth but ignoring
the postpartum period the first time around; second-timers
often think less about the birth and more about what follows

it. The best advice I can think to give is to imagine that you will be a person of great significance after you give birth; channel your inner Aphrodite, the goddess of fertility, who herself was a mother and so would have known how it felt to bleed from her nipples or get a wet patch in her pants whenever she sneezed. You should be waited on, pampered, listened to and comforted whenever you feel sad. And you may need your partner, midwife, friend or family member to help you get extra healthcare or support. Don't fall into the trap of trying to 'bounce back', as the trope goes. Relish recovering slowly. And plan for how that's going to happen. If you can face it, read ahead to Part 3 and beyond, but for starters, make sure you have plenty of maternity pads, loose and comfortable clothing, soft and supportive pillows, multivitamins and nutritious snacks and drinks as well as fresh and frozen food. Think about your support network – who is going to help you and when – and make sure you use it. And get ready to be selfish; you may want to limit visitors and embrace the intimacy of your new family, or just remind yourself that there's no need to cater for other people as you would have done before.

Lily Nichols, American dietician/nutritionist and author of Real Food for Pregnancy, *on her postpartum recovery:*
'I felt really, really well prepared for pregnancy and then postpartum was like, wow. I was unprepared for the amount of time it would take for your body to recover; the massive increase in appetite was a surprise; the months of sleep disruption; how long it takes for your pelvic floor to return. I tried to go out for a hike at two months postpartum. No, no, no, my friend – recovery takes a long time! My second

postpartum recovery, however, was smooth as silk because I didn't have all these unrealistic expectations.'

Should you eat your placenta?

Hilary Duff whizzed hers up and had it in a smoothie. Alicia Silverstone took hers in one pill a day – her 'happy pill', as her husband called it. Kim Kardashian did the same. The list of celebrities who have allegedly consumed their own placentas grows ever longer, leaving the rest of us to wonder what we're missing out on.

Women who eat their placenta argue that the iron and protein it contains help the body recover, and that consuming it can ward off depression, improve milk supply and stop bleeding. Another argument commonly deployed is that almost all other mammals – apart from camels – have been seen to eat theirs, so surely it follows that we should too. The trouble is, however, there is no research to back up any of this.

Timothy Caulfield is a health law professor at the University of Alberta in Canada and author of *Is Gwyneth Paltrow Wrong About Everything?* In an interview, printed in *Scientific American,* he says that eating your placenta has absolutely no documented health benefits. Caulfield describes it as a classic example of people doing something just because celebrities do it. 'The power of celebrity culture is profound, and I really think this is an example of it,' he said.

While there is no evidence in favour of placentophagy, as it's called, there is one alarming case against it. In 2016, a baby born in Oregon was quickly diagnosed with a strep infection, which meant it had trouble breathing. After antibiotics, the baby was diagnosed with exactly the same infection a second time. Luckily, doctors were quick to work out that the mother was taking placenta pills. They tested the pills and found that they were the source of the infection. A report published by the US Centers for Disease Control and Prevention said that the pills had likely increased the number of strep bacteria in the mother's intestine and skin, from which the baby picked up the infection.

So there you have it: why Kim Kardashian thinks you should eat your placenta, and why the US Centers for Disease Control and Prevention thinks you shouldn't. If you do decide to ingest yours, you'll find recipes online – placenta chilli, for example – or you can arrange for it to be collected, freeze-dried and sent back to you in capsule form by one of the private placenta encapsulation companies who offer the service in the UK.

3

During Birth

Almost every pregnant woman wants her baby's birth to be uncomplicated, and we write birth plans that reflect that. Unfortunately, however, our bodies and babies don't always get the memo, which is why some obstetricians discourage pregnant women, particularly first-timers, from writing detailed birth plans. But choosing not to write a birth plan doesn't mean you shouldn't prepare for labour. While your baby's safe delivery will, of course, be your primary concern, know that there are a few key things that are shown to minimise the impact of a vaginal birth on your body.

Hands-on birth

If you have a vaginal birth, you'll want a midwife to support your perineum (the layers of muscle between your vagina and back passage) as the baby's head comes out, to manage its exit and prevent tearing. The midwife typically controls the delivery of the baby's head with her left hand while her right hand supports the perineum.

Warm perineal compress

Warm things stretch better, which is why the World Health Organization recommends your midwife or doctor puts a warm compress on your perineum as the baby is crowning, to reduce tearing.

Ventouse versus forceps: know the difference

There are three reasons why you might need either a ventouse or forceps delivery: because your baby is not coming out of the birth canal as expected, because there are concerns about its wellbeing, or because you are unable to, or have been told not to, push. Forceps are smooth, curved, metal instruments, like tongs, that fit around your baby's head and, when you have a contraction, are used to help to pull the baby out. A ventouse is a suction cup that attaches to the baby's head by creating a vacuum and also helps to pull it out, a bit like a plumber's plunger.

Having your baby delivered with forceps poses a greater risk to your short- and long-term pelvic floor health than a ventouse delivery does. In the US, Germany, Sweden and Denmark, forceps deliveries are now rare; they account for less than 0.5 per cent of deliveries. Instead, where possible, doctors use ventouse suction caps, which result in less tearing and don't always need an episiotomy.

Forceps are more successful than a ventouse suction cap, however, which is why there is a place for them. The choice of ventouse versus forceps depends on numerous factors, including pain relief, your baby's wellbeing and the position of its head. If the fetus is showing signs of distress and a rapid delivery is required, forceps may be more appropriate. Or, if the woman hasn't been able to push well and there is no sign of fetal distress, the ventouse may be more appropriate. The doctor's choice may also be guided by his or her experience and training.

Whatever happens, your reasons for needing an assisted birth and the proposed method should be explained to you by your obstetrician or midwife beforehand, and you will need to give verbal consent. If a ventouse is not discussed, don't be afraid to ask why; it's vital that you feel informed and comfortable with whatever decision you make. And, if your doctor or midwife is making you uncomfortable, you are within your rights to ask for someone else.

Focus on the push, relax the jaw

When I was busy with the final push, the midwives kept telling me to relax my jaw. It was not the time to ask why, so I did what I was told, never quite understanding it. At the time, I assumed they were just trying to get me to focus all my energy and attention on the push, rather than on my jaw. Reading about it later, however, I discovered that there is a documented connection between the jaw and the pelvic floor, and that releasing one can simultaneously release the other. Both areas respond to emotions and stress; the connection is perhaps most obvious in dogs, who set their jaws, bare their teeth and clamp their tails when stressed, but pant, loll their tongues and wag their tails when content. If you've done pelvic floor training or hypnobirthing, you may not need midwives to tell you to relax your jaw in order to release your pelvic floor – but it's worth considering, as it may help.

Rectal exam after vaginal birth

In an attempt to improve identification of third- and fourth-degree tears, obstetricians and gynaecologists have been piloting new measures, including a rectal exam after every vaginal birth to ensure no damage to the back passage goes unseen. It involves – you guessed it – a quick finger up the bum, and it is already part of the normal routine for obstetricians after they repair tears. A missed tear into the anus can lead to devastating consequences, including long-term faecal incontinence. Despite the initial success of this pilot and plans to roll out routine rectal exams across the country, many midwives haven't heard of this. If your midwife doesn't offer it, you can request one after the birth to ensure they haven't missed anything.

Get whatever you need to feel safe

Women in labour want to be treated with care, consideration and expertise. Sadly, this isn't always the case. Between 25 and 34 per cent of women in the UK report that their birth was traumatic. It's not *what* happens to you in clinical terms that causes birth trauma, but your *experience* of it. As one midwife told me, plenty of women have ideal births on paper but are traumatised because of how the people around them made them feel. Knowing this, trauma experts recommend you choose where you give birth, and your birth partner, carefully. Who makes you feel safest? Assuming it's your husband or partner, consider what level of involvement they will be comfortable with. Make sure they understand what you want and need and are ready to advocate for you, and don't be afraid to ask questions of your midwives or doctors. They should assess your individual risk and be able to advise you on where it is safest for you to deliver. As hypnobirthing studies prove, your mindset – in particular how safe you feel – is important to how well you give birth and may influence your choice. Ultimately, however, it's the doctors and midwives who will likely guide you towards an informed decision, based on your personal history and decades of medical research.

> *Alex Heath, a clinical hypnotherapist specialising in birth trauma, advises that you decide where you feel safest, who's going to support you best, then prepare:*
> 'The way to avoid trauma is to feel very, very safe. Ask yourself, where will I feel safest – in a hospital, or at home? That is a major consideration. And then you need to gather your team around you – and that is not always your partner, unfortunately. You need to have that conversation, and say, this is what I need from you on the day. I think there's a great strength in discussing that and acknowledging it. You need to dig deep into yourself and say, how will I feel most safe and supported? And you need to prepare – whether through antenatal courses, working with a doula, doing an online course or listening to hypnosis audio recordings.'

My birth story

I went into labour ten days late, after my seventh curry, walk, pineapple and sexual undertaking in as many days. We played backgammon (I won) then went to bed, and it was just after I turned off the light that I felt my first contractions, like period pains. They were around seven minutes apart and I snuck out of bed to leave Philip to get some sleep. By 2.30 a.m., I could no longer be quiet. I needed to make noise. So I sat on the side of the bed and gently woke him. By 5.30 a.m., the contractions felt strong. I didn't want to deliver on the bathroom floor, so we went to the hospital. They examined me, and suggested I go home. A measly one centimetre. The knock to my pride didn't put me off, however, and when we got home, it became a blur; by late morning, I was definitely in active labour. Philip tried to persuade me to eat some Marmite on toast as I spread across the back seat of the car, moaning, as we drove back again. (I'd asked him to make sure I ate to keep my strength up – marathon training – but had a sudden aversion to food.)

They didn't need to examine me at the hospital: I'd had one contraction in the revolving door, another in the lift, and a third as we got to the reception. Once in the birthing suite, things calmed down – which was normal, according to our midwife. After a few hours I was back in the zone, demanding gas and air whenever I felt a contraction coming with the intensity of an addict. In between contractions, Philip poked crumbs of flapjack into my mouth, and we giggled as he tried the laughing gas – but I quickly turned formidable when I felt another surge coming on and demanded it back.

The midwife sat around a corner, getting on with some paperwork and coming to examine me every hour or so. By half-past five, I was fully dilated and ready to push, but the contractions dried up. The baby was calm, but at some point the nurses started to talk about breaking my waters or getting me onto the labour ward for a syntocinon – synthetic hormone – drip.

Keen to avoid intervention, my husband and I ramped up the experimentation. A new midwife entered the room to find me circling my hips intently and Philip diligently tweaking both nipples from behind like he was tuning an old radio. I lunged, I squatted, I hula'd, but not much changed. In a flight of genius, Philip thought to change the music. One of our favourite albums by a friend's band had been on for a while, and it was sombre and brooding, like Radiohead.

Philip switched it for something more upbeat and suddenly we were back on track. I pushed, and pushed, in all manner of positions, swore a lot, and finally my waters broke, sending a midwife diving out of the way. The baby was coming, but still took its time. Finally, at 7.30 p.m., the promise of one last push turned out to be true.

Part 2

THE FIRST SIX WEEKS

Waking as a mother for the first time, my initial thought was one of deep and fulsome joy, that we had a healthy baby boy. My second was that I couldn't sit up to look at him. My core muscles – so-called because they form the literal core of your body and you're not good for much without them – were gone. When I rolled over and tried to bring the baby, which weighed no more than your average cat, towards me, I couldn't do that either.

I thought childbirth would be the end of the months of physical upheaval. But, after spending weeks wishing the baby out and pregnancy over, it turned out to be just the beginning. At 34, I'd just got used to a body with a finite list of functions, a certain hormone profile and a mostly stable shape, and then overnight my nipples became a source of sustenance, my form underwent a complete metamorphosis and my hormone levels made the 2008 stock market crash look like a gentle decline.

The spectrum of what recovery looks like for a woman after birth is huge, ranging from those who are fine to go for a gentle jog after two weeks (see Chapter 18) to those who stay in bed for a month or more. The first six weeks, known medically as the puerperium, is the time it takes your genitals and pelvic organs to migrate back to something approaching their starting position. This process is largely the same for all of us: the cervix closes, the uterus shrinks, your abdominal muscles knit back together and the rest of your organs breathe a sigh of relief. You are now in a new state of normal. But while most of us experience these changes in a similar way, our experience of everything else is wildly unpredictable.

When I did eventually achieve a sitting position by rolling onto my side and pushing myself up with my hands, I became aware of the pain down below. Whether it was the graze on my vagina, or the general trauma of pushing a baby through an opening designed to accommodate a penis, it was made worse by the absorbent pad that had buckled up into uncomfortable ridges during the night.

We'd chosen to come home soon after the birth, around midnight, so there were no midwives on hand to tell us what to do. After persuading the baby to suckle on colostrum, Philip and I located a book someone had given us that provided a week-by-week account of life with a newborn. 'Week one ...' It's astonishing that you don't have to pass a test before being left in sole charge of a baby. Deliriously happy, but also startled and wide-eyed at our rapid change in circumstances, we tried our best to read attentively whilst sitting up in bed drinking tea.

My next personal revelation came only after I'd had some breakfast and discovered that I was unable to hold a fart. When I tried to tense my pelvic floor, it seemed that the muscles had taken leave of my body completely, together with my core. But rather than embrace my delicate and enfeebled state by staying in bed and being waited on, I ignored it. By the end of the first week, I had been to the pub for lunch, gone out for a walk and shared more than one bottle of champagne (albeit just a small glass of each). By the end of the second week, we'd had friends over for dinner, I was regularly out with the baby, and I'd even taken on some work. At the start of the third week, we dutifully opened our week-by-week baby book to see what we should be doing now. Both Philip and I stopped in disbelief at the first line: 'You may now be thinking about leaving the house for the first time.' Eh?

I was a poster child for the modern have-it-all woman, and a fool for being proud of it. We are brought up in a system that values everything but torpor and incapacity. Women have battled the patriarchy for a hundred years, and we've won so much – but we have lost our ability to embrace moments of weakness and vulnerability. As the Harvard Professor of Government Harvey Mansfield says, there is a contradiction at the heart of feminism: 'Women are no longer the weaker sex, but they remain the more vulnerable sex,' and yet vulnerability is the contrary of independence. Take strength from embracing your vulnerability for a while. Take your recovery seriously; try to focus on nothing but feeding the baby, resting, sleeping and eating; be kind to your body, and take all the help you can get. Rather than attempt to look and act like someone who hasn't just had a baby, enjoy being someone who has.

Before we get into the details of recovery, there are a few things that everyone needs to know:

Moving around – Women used to be strictly confined to bed after birth but are now encouraged to move around little and often, to improve circulation, promote healing and prevent blood clots.

Lifting – Try to avoid lifting anything heavier than your baby during the first six weeks, but don't berate yourself if you do need to. How you lift is more important than what you lift, so bend your knees, keep your back straight and pull your abdominal muscles in towards your spine. And use a pram rather than carry your baby around in a car seat, if you can.

Driving – If you've had a caesarean, the NHS recommends that you don't drive for the first six weeks, but this doesn't mean everyone should get back behind the wheel at that point. In legal terms, you can drive as soon as you feel in control, can do an emergency stop and your insurance has no clause that exempts you from doing so. But it's advised that you exercise caution, even if you do feel up to it; having to brake sharply, for example, could cause you undue pain as it overwhelms your recovering muscles. When you do get back behind the wheel, a cushion on your belly may make the seatbelt more comfortable against your scar.

Exercise – After six weeks, you should be able to start swimming again and do low-impact exercise like walking. The NHS recommends that you wait until at least 12 weeks to resume high-impact exercise like running and CrossFit. Physiotherapists caution that this is too soon for many women;

they say you should wait for up to six months if you've had a caesarean, episiotomy, significant tearing or muscle damage. Physios urge you to go for an assessment if there's anything that doesn't feel right, but also if you're asymptomatic; they say that any postpartum woman planning a return to high-impact exercise, including running, should get checked out first. Somewhere along this spectrum of advice lies what's right for you (see Chapter 18 for more).

4

Vaginal Birth Recovery

When I first tried to flex the muscles around my vagina, urethra and rectum, it was like I had the opposite of phantom limb syndrome – I knew the right muscles were there, they had to be, but I felt nothing at all. In exchange, I seemed to have acquired an entirely new body part, one that existed prior to birth, but which I had never been regularly aware of before: my vagina, or 'frankengina', as one friend fondly called hers. As that friend said to me, in the weeks after birth it was so tender and out of shape that she encountered it all the time. 'Oh, hello vagina ... Oh, there you go again,' she would think, as it made itself known to her throughout the day.

No matter how well your birth went, you'll be sore down under. If your nerves have been stretched and damaged, you may also be missing some vital functions, such as the muscles that once controlled your bladder and bowel; and you might have piles, amongst other delights. Try to talk openly with your midwife (and partner) so you're not hiding things, and don't worry – all of this is common to start with, and normal functioning should return.

Having avoided drugs during pregnancy, I initially forgot that I could take painkillers to make it all more bearable; even if you're breastfeeding you can take the maximum dosage of paracetamol and ibuprofen, either together or at overlapping intervals, if you need to.

Vagina and vulva

I'd never heard the word 'dragging' in any context other than moving uncooperative objects and people around – until I gave birth. Dragging commonly refers to the bulging or heaviness you may feel inside and outside your vagina, in the lower abdomen, or around your back passage, after birth. Often, it seems much worse to you than it looks to someone else. If you've ever had any issues with body dysmorphia, it's common to develop a distorted view of how your vagina and vulva look. Numbness is also common at the start, due to the nerves having been stretched; it's a traction injury, Kate Walsh at Liverpool Women's Hospital explains, and nerves can take months, and sometimes years, to heal.

What to expect

Physios say you should expect the area around your vagina to look more 'frilly' than usual immediately after birth, perhaps with skin tags where they didn't use to be. The vulva is always open after birth, like it's yawning. At the back of the vaginal opening, the perineum might no longer be so clearly defined because the vaginal opening has stretched. You may be able to see ridges of the vagina (that are usually hidden) down at the entrance, which can make you think it's a prolapse. Your anus will likely be bulging and engorged (and can stay like that for some time). You may also see a scar, if you had an episiotomy or tear, and stitches. Scars can be very sensitive long after they've healed, so the advice is that, once it's healed, you should touch and massage it regularly.

These changes will disappear with time, but some things will never go back to exactly how they were, a fact that most women come to terms with. You've done something miraculous, after all, and a little cosmetic change is entirely natural and nothing to worry about. The pressure on us to look a certain way, however, is getting worse – more and more women are having surgery to correct changes to their vulvas after childbirth – but even in this day and age few can claim the need for an Instagrammable vagina. It can help to see any asymptomatic changes that result from childbirth, such as skin tags, stretch marks or slightly separated abdominal muscles, as adaptations rather than injuries. If something isn't affecting your body's functioning, then it's up to you whether you see it as an injury, which is negative, or an adaptation, which is positive, and testament to your body's extraordinary ability to change.

Vulval varicosities

These darlings – the vagina's version of a haemorrhoid, if you will – crop up in around 20 per cent of pregnant women. Often, it feels like you have very swollen genitals, with pain that gets worse after sex, standing or physical activity. In around 95 per cent of cases, they usually disappear within six weeks of birth, or shrivel up leaving just small skin tags. (If they don't, a surgical procedure can remove them.)

Dry skin

Having dry lady bits is a common cause of postpartum pain. As described in Part 1, hormones whose levels peak during the third trimester – notably oestrogen and progesterone – plummet after you give birth, and the drop in oestrogen means that your skin is often dry for a while afterwards. And when skin gets dry, it gets sore – including your most sensitive tissue, which has been on a rollercoaster of ups and downs recently.

Kate Walsh recommends 'v-acials' – like facials, but for the vulva, which involve regularly moisturising and massaging the vulva and perineum. 'I've had women who feel that they may have developed a prolapse when often it's poor-quality skin creating that sensation,' she says, and all they need to do is moisturise and improve the condition of the tissues.

Don't use any old moisturiser, though. You can use a proprietary moisturiser (Kate recommends one made by the 'organic intimacy company' YES, which is also available on prescription through the NHS), or just a natural moisturiser like coconut or almond oil. Going further, Kate suggests we consider treating postnatal women as we do menopausal women, since both are oestrogen-depleted, by replenishing their vaginas (after they finish breastfeeding) with topical oestrogen treatments to perk them up again. Oestrogen gels are currently prescribed for vaginal dryness caused by menopausal changes – known as hormone replacement therapy, or HRT – but perhaps such a super-charged 'v-acial' for postpartum women including a dose of oestrogen lies not too far away in the future.

Monitoring your healing

The trouble with monitoring our recovery from a vaginal birth is that many of us didn't know what our vaginas and vulvas looked like in the first place. Generations of women before us have done anything to avoid saying the word vulva, glossed over the female anatomy, and taught us to feel awkward about our lady parts. Now is the time to know and become comfortable with yours.

If you're unsure about how you're healing, it's important that someone (yourself included) takes a look. It is common to feel embarrassed, or reluctant to invite yet more invasions of your private life, but the benefits of professional reassurance should outweigh any discomfort you feel. With hindsight, I'd have greatly preferred a midwife to examine my healing vagina rather than, as it turned out, my husband.

I had voiced concerns about my graze and general healing on a number of occasions in the days after the birth, but I had never asked my midwife to look. One evening, Philip tackled the problem head-on.

'Right. Knickers down, knees up,' he commanded.

'What, me?' I yelped.

'Yes. I think it's important to know how it's healing.'

Crikey. The last time his head went this far south it was... well, quite another thing. I prevaricated and tried to dissuade him, but he would not be put off. He ignored my protestations and – poof – just like that, another of our boundaries went up in smoke. Afterwards, I felt immensely better that he had seen it, reassured me, and not run away.

Too often, women take on their healing as yet another thing they have to sort out themselves, rather than something they allow their partner to share or support them with. You've got to allow them the chance to help. If that's not something you're comfortable with, ask your midwife or a doctor to take a look – or anyone you trust. With no one else available, one friend of mine even asked her mother-in-law to examine her – and was glad that she did so. Don't be afraid to go to your midwife, GP, hospital or nearest perineal trauma clinic if instinct tells you something isn't right. If there is a problem that hasn't been spotted, such as a missed tear or infection, the sooner it's treated, the better.

Grazes, cuts, tears and stitches

The body has an amazing ability to recover from insults, but there is something about an injury in a woman's genitalia that can leave her feeling intensely, uniquely vulnerable; even a minor graze can make every movement agony and be a constant reminder of the wound. You may feel bruised, as well, both emotionally and physically. One woman I interviewed felt let down by the fact that she'd torn, even though it was only minor. 'I hated the fact that I hadn't had control and blamed the midwives for not telling me to stop pushing,' she recalls. If you had an episiotomy with a forceps or ventouse delivery, or sustained a significant tear, and didn't feel well supported, you might feel angry, remorseful or disappointed. Ensure you are waited on for a couple of weeks. Surround yourself with pillows and find positions that work for you. You also need to take great care to prevent infection, and look out for signs that one is developing. (See page 74 for advice on monitoring your wound.) The cut or tear should heal within a few weeks, but the stitches might feel itchy as the wound is healing. You may also see stitches falling out when it has healed, which is normal.

The First Six Weeks

First-degree tears

These are small tears or grazes that only affect the skin, either around the labia, clitoris or inside the vagina. They usually resolve quickly without treatment and don't cause any long-term symptoms, but they can be very sore until they heal. (See page 79 for tips on making yourself comfortable.)

Second-degree tears

Going slightly deeper than first-degree tears, these affect the skin and the perineal muscle and usually require stitches. You were probably repaired in the room where you gave birth under local anaesthetic and are unlikely to have any long-term symptoms, although the healing process can be incredibly sore. A severe second-degree tear could really be a misdiagnosed third-degree tear, however (see below), so talk to your midwife or doctor if you're worried that there is damage to your back passage or elsewhere. You may need additional care, including physiotherapy, to support your recovery.

Third- and fourth-degree tears

Known as OASIs (obstetric anal sphincter injuries), these are serious injuries where a tear through the muscle of your perineum extends into your back passage. They affect 7 per cent of women during their first labour, and 2 per cent of those who have given birth previously, but there is evidence to show that many more OASIs are missed. Although now out of date, a paper from 1993 revealed that 35 per cent of first-time mums in the UK showed evidence of anal sphincter injury using diagnostic ultrasound, and the injury was

64

still there at six months postpartum (although only a third of them had symptoms). Since then, rates of recognised OASIs have more than doubled, but this could be due to better identification, and recovery is generally good, especially if the tear is identified and repaired quickly. Obstetricians note, however, that it's not always possible to identify sphincter injuries immediately after birth, so it's important to properly investigate if there are any ongoing problems. If you have had an OASI repair, you should expect to see a physiotherapist before leaving hospital and again afterwards, to check how it's healing.

Everyone's recovery will look different but it's normal to feel pain for up to three weeks, especially when walking or sitting – so most of the time. It's possible that the sphincter is weaker or doesn't heal properly, in which case you may have some leaking of wind and/or small amounts of poo. And you might fart more easily or have to rush to get to the loo in time. You will need to go back to the specialist urogynaecology clinic for a follow-up appointment, but if you're worried, call the clinic or ask to see your doctor. If you're still experiencing incontinence or pain at your follow-up appointment, guidelines state that you should be referred to a specialist gynaecologist or colorectal surgeon. That won't necessarily mean you need more surgery – you may just need physiotherapy. Guidelines state that you should also receive psychological support if it has affected your mental health, but it's not always offered, so push for it if you want it. The MASIC Foundation (a catchy acronym for Mothers with Anal Sphincter Injuries in Childbirth) also organises support groups and provides a lot of information online for mums with an OASI (see Resources).

Lisa Cornwell, mum of two and blogger at mumma-scribbles.com, had an episiotomy with her second child (a vaginal birth after a caesarean), so doctors could use a ventouse cap and forceps to help the baby out:

'I didn't know why I was in so much pain until I was brave and looked down there to see that the whole area was black and blue. The fact that I couldn't sit down made complete sense at that point! For the first week, I was basically lying down; moving to a standing position was incredibly painful. Into the second week, the bruising had started to go down and I could start to sit up a bit more for short periods. I honestly had no idea that this would be the case, however, so it was a bit of a shock to the system. I'm not going to lie – the pain has been immense and for me the recovery has been comparable to that of a C-section. This has really upset me at times because one of the biggest reasons I didn't want a C-section was so that I could be up and about quickly, but sadly I have spent most of my other half's two weeks off laid up on the sofa, struggling to get up and walk around and feeling utterly useless. He was changing all of the nappies, handing me the baby when he needed feeding, cleaning, looking after our baby, etc. He was amazing and I hope that you get the level of support I have had because you really do need it.'

Managing stitches

Stitches should start healing after five days, but midwives say the wound can take up to 21 days to heal as multiple layers of tissue may need to knit back together. In between the individual stitches, it might feel like you still have an extra hole or two. There is no need to panic. Your body is busy repairing the wound from the inside out, so it will take a while to heal over completely and, as it does so, it may feel like you have little gaps in between. The wound may also bleed.

Keeping your perineum clean is easier said than done, given all of the bodily fluids that are in the mix, plus the fact that you're constantly wearing a pad. One friend would sit on a disposable incontinence sheet without knickers to air it (see page 79). Wash the area gently as often as you like, but try to give it a good wash daily – either a sitz bath, a proper bath or a shower. You can put tea tree oil in your bath as this has antibacterial properties, and let it disperse through the water with a glug of milk (which stops the oil floating on the surface) – but don't use salt until the wound has healed as it can dissolve the stitches too quickly. You can also use a peri-bottle (see page 150) or keep a jug of water in the bathroom that you pour over yourself after you use the loo. It's vital that you dry it well because a moist environment encourages bacteria. Use loo roll or a towel, provided it's clean. Change your pads frequently; midwives advise using cotton-based ones (often called 'maternity pads') rather than those made from plastic, which they claim can lead to infection.

Going to the loo can be daunting (see page 148). Avoid constipation at all costs; if you have stitches, your doctor may have prescribed a laxative, but if not you should increase your fibre intake or supplement your diet with a stool softener such as Dulcolease, or soaked or ground linseed to prevent straining on the loo.

Infections

No matter what precautions you take, it's possible that you might get an infection through no fault of your own – sometimes from bacteria that was there when your wound was repaired. The area might smell bad, be red, warm and inflamed, increasingly painful and tender, or you might feel unwell with a fever, chills, pain in the lower abdomen and cramping. Contact your midwife straight away if you think you might have an infection.

> *Cassia, 34, a mother of two, had an episiotomy with her second birth, a vaginal birth after caesarean (VBAC). After five days, midwives said she had 'a slight infection':* 'I'd had a massive episiotomy and then all the stitches dissolved because the infection was so bad. My instant reaction was, is it because I haven't been keeping it clean? But the midwife explained it wasn't that and it's really common. I feel like it needed to be more deeply cleaned before I was stitched up – but my legs were in the air, I couldn't see a thing. And there's the blood that's constantly coming out of you – it's moist and warm the whole time, which is the perfect set-up for an infection. I had to wait four weeks to have it redone under general anaesthetic and had six layers of stitches put in. It was so bad they wanted a senior surgeon to do it, and they also wanted to make sure the infection had completely cleared up. Afterwards, I was concerned the same thing might happen again, even though they'd done six layers. You do hear of cases where the hospitals say they don't re-stitch; one friend was told it would just gradually heal with time. The experience affected me a lot. As I tried to put it to my husband, how would you feel if you were walking around with your dick split in two? He's been amazing, but then I don't think a man can fully appreciate what it's like to have something like that. It affected me far more than what was a much more scary situation with my first born's emergency C-section. The way I was left feeling mutilated was horrid.*

*When I look at pictures of my daughter when she was a baby
I have this underlying urge to wince; I even clench my bottom.
It was such a happy time, but it was tinged with this awful
experience. For a good while afterwards I thought I would
definitely not have any more children; I love both my children so much but I thought, I can't put my body through this
again. Now, when we talk about having another child, it's a
massive factor for me, and that's something I think is very
hard for lots of men to understand. It's just such a personal
part of your body. It frustrates me that the NHS would say
that it was a "successful" VBAC delivery. I couldn't walk for
six weeks.'*

Managing pain

Physios say that you should sit as little as possible while your
wound is healing (around eight days), because sitting tends
to stretch the pelvic floor and decrease blood flow to the
pelvic area. For when you do need to sit, you can get ring-
shaped cushions to help with the pain, so that your vulva
doesn't make contact with whatever you're sitting on – but
these bum doughnuts are controversial. Firstly, some level
of compression – though not always comfortable – is actually helpful because it supports the pelvic floor, minimising
stretching. That's why, if you do need to sit, a stable exercise
ball is a good idea, or just a set of pillows. If a doughnut is
what best works for you, however, don't beat yourself up –
do what you need to get by. Whatever happens, just don't let
your sitting position put undue pressure on your stitches;
make sure you're not pulling them apart.

Padsicles

It's becoming popular to make 'padsicles' – frozen pads that you put in your pants to promote healing. There is limited evidence to suggest they speed up healing – a 2012 Cochrane Review found no evidence for this – but there is some evidence to show that using ice packs can reduce the pain after giving birth. This is backed up by sports scientists, who say that ice helps with pain but not tissue repair, and by the many women who say it feels good. To try one, soak a thick sanitary pad in water and place it in the freezer. Thaw it for five to ten minutes before putting it into your pants. Warning: it will defrost fairly quickly, so either sit on a towel or use another pad or even some incontinence pants over it. Some people suggest adding witch hazel and/or aloe vera, which you can if you like, although, again, evidence for its efficacy is limited. You can also buy reusable cold pads, which may be less messy. Or improvise with the old classic: a bag of frozen peas and a tea towel.

5

Caesarean Recovery

Caesarean sections account for more than a quarter of births in the UK and are the most-commonly performed major operation in the world. In spite of this, many childbirth classes make only passing mention of them, and the procedure is rarely shown in films or on television, leaving many women to feel underprepared; too often, we are sold a fairy tale of 'natural' childbirth when we live in a modern world. Women who have emergency caesareans can sometimes feel that they have somehow failed, but a woman who gives birth via caesarean has still given birth, which is an incomparable achievement. And the choices that she and her doctors made were absolutely the right ones if both she and the baby are OK.

A caesarean involves a huge and rapid physiological shift. If it was unplanned, you may have also felt out of control, with mounting levels of fear or stress. An emergency caesarean is linked to higher rates of postnatal depression and post-traumatic stress disorder, so pay attention to your mental health in these early weeks.

It's impossible to predict how quickly you'll be up and about but you should expect a significant period of rest and recovery. Multiple layers of tissue have been cut and sewn back together, meaning multiple layers of tissue have to heal. It could take weeks, or it could take months, depending on

The mother of all caesareans

In 1809, a time when women were not allowed to be doctors, a young Irishwoman living in London called Margaret Bulkley was so determined to enter the profession that she disguised herself as a man. Her uncle paid for her to go to medical school, where her petite build was attributed to her young age. She adopted the name James Barry, after her now late-uncle, and returned to London a qualified doctor. As a member of the Royal College of Surgeons, she joined the British Army and for the next 50 years served all over the world, becoming a celebrated surgeon and pioneer of surgical techniques. She conducted the first successful caesarean in Cape Town in 1826. Not once did anyone publicly question her gender; people simply did not consider a woman capable of being a doctor at that time. When Margaret – or James – died in 1865, her request that she be buried without examination was not heeded. The woman preparing the corpse discovered that James was a woman and, even more unbelievably, found stretch marks from a pregnancy. It later emerged that she had been raped in her youth and given birth to a baby, which her mother had raised.

any complications and whether you have other demands on you. Some women report feeling back to normal within a week or two, but doctors warn that your body may trick you into thinking you're healed, and then you do too much too soon, which will set back your recovery.

The first week: the basics

When you get out of bed, roll onto your side first and push yourself up with your arms to a sitting position. Do the reverse when getting back into bed. If lying flat pulls on your scar at all, you can put a cushion under your knees (if you lie on your back) or under your tummy (if you lie on your side). When lying down or sitting, shift your position regularly to avoid getting stiff or sore.

It's recommended that you get up and walk around a little soon after a caesarean – the same day, if you can. Physios admit that this sounds a bit mad, but it helps to manage the swelling and pain. Trapped wind can actually be more painful than the scar, and movement also helps with this (as does peppermint tea).

When walking, think about your posture and try to keep your body upright. Even going from a sitting to a standing position exerts a significant amount of pressure on your abdomen, so move gently.

If you cough, sneeze or laugh, try to bend your knees up and support your incision with your hands, a cushion or a towel (unless you're wearing a belly bind – see page 157 for more). And if your legs and ankles are swollen, elevate them, point your toes and rotate your ankles regularly.

Go to the loo every two to three hours because, due to the effects of the anaesthetic, your bladder might not tell you when it's full for up to a week after your caesarean. If you struggle to get to the loo in time or don't think your bladder is emptying properly, contact your midwife. A pelvic health physio should be able to help if your midwife can't. Trapped wind can present as pain in your stomach or shoulder. To help it leave your body, you can massage your tummy with a clockwise motion whilst supporting your stitches, try to move around little and often, bend your knees and put your feet on the bed then move the knees from left to right, and drink peppermint tea (or the medicinal version, peppermint water).

A lot of women experience constipation, which can feel alarming. Deep breathing, and moving around little and often, can help to prevent it. (See page 151 for more on how to manage this.)

Wound care

A horizontal incision is now used in 95 per cent of caesareans. It cuts across the bottom of the uterus, where it is thinnest, to minimise bleeding, and it is less likely than other types of incision to split in the future. A vertical incision is used only when necessary and results in a vertical scar from the tummy button downwards. It might hurt a little more and heal more slowly than a horizontal incision.

Either way, you'll have a dressing covering the wound for at least 24 hours. Once it's removed, keep the wound clean and dry, washing it gently with warm water – it's enough to let soapy water pass over it in the shower – once a day. Air the scar as much as possible because it will speed up the healing. You don't need to be naked – just wear a loose cotton shirt or dress at night and something similar in the day. After a week or so it might start to itch, which shows it's healing.

Some stitches require removal, others dissolve; you should be told which sort yours are. If you have the dissolvable kind and your wound has healed but your stitches haven't gone, you can book an appointment with a nurse or GP to remove them. Some women experience minor infections, discomfort or unusual scar tissue if the stitches are left there for too long.

Meg's baby, who was born with a rare condition called Congenital Diaphragmatic Hernia, was born by caesarean, before undergoing an operation that saved his life: 'I love my scar, and because my baby was poorly he has a scar too. I love that we have our own scars and our own story.'

Scar tissue massage

Research shows that massage can help to soften and flatten scar tissue, reduce pain and improve normal sensation around the area of the caesarean wound. It can also help with the muscle recovery, pulling and tightness.

Once your incision has healed, usually after three to six weeks, soft-tissue experts suggest you start by moving your hands in a circular motion over your belly so that you feel gentle pulling sensations on the scar tissue below. By moving the top layer of skin around, you'll also be moving the top layer of connective tissue, which can loosen up any tight spots and generate heat and extra blood flow to speed up healing.

After that, you can start massaging the area immediately around the scar. Lie flat on your back so your muscles are relaxed and use two fingers to massage the skin in a circular motion, 20 to 30 times. Again, you're aiming to move the skin, not to draw circles on top of it. If you find a spot where it's tight, work on it.

You can also use an oil like vitamin E or coconut to massage the scar directly. Physiotherapists recommend you make small circles over the scar itself, slowly increasing the amount of pressure as it is comfortable to do so.

The First Six Weeks

Infection

Normal healing involves slight redness along the wound, possibly some swelling and pain, and a small amount of clear fluid coming out. Signs of a possible infection include increasing redness, heat, swelling or tenderness (especially if you feel it when you're resting), a change in the colour, volume or smell of the fluid coming from the wound, having a temperature and feeling generally unwell.

The NHS recommends that you shouldn't use tampons or menstrual cups until you've had your six-week check. There is no rule about when you can have sex, but wait at least a few weeks and until you feel fully comfortable. Your body is open to infection at various sites after giving birth, which means it is more vulnerable than usual; you don't want any bacteria travelling up through your cervix.

Maria still feels occasional twinges in her incision over two years on:
'I remember finding the stinging really tough, especially at night when you suddenly go from a relaxed, deep sleep into the pain of moving. But it's amazing how quickly my core came back. Over time, the hardest thing I found was that it ached whenever I ran after giving birth. That went on for over a year. Even sometimes when I do weights now, more than two years on, I get a little stinging pain. It takes time to fully heal.'

6

Cramping and Bleeding

Postpartum bleeding is an inconvenience that no one prepared me for. I knew I would lose blood immediately afterwards – around half a litre after a vaginal birth, and a litre after a C-section, by all accounts – but it just kept coming. The word for this is lochia, taken from the Greek word *Lokhia*, meaning childbirth, and it's like a long, heavy period that can contain a beguiling mix of substances including baby poo, vernix (the cheesy protective layer) and lanugo (the light fur that covers babies in the womb), as well as the more predictable blood and tissue.

Whether you gave birth vaginally or by C-section, you will have a large wound inside you where the placenta used to attach to the womb. As this and other tissues heal, you will experience bleeding that can last up to six weeks; it is typically heavy for only the first week or ten days, then it should decrease in volume and colour over time.

Initially, lochia should be red and smell earthy or fleshy, and this stage will last three to seven days. If it starts to smell funny, ask a healthcare provider to take a look as you could have an infection (see page 80). Passing clots is completely normal, and they can be huge without being cause for concern – up to the size of a golf ball according to the NHS (for anything larger than that, see page 80.)

Disconcertingly, you may find you bleed more when you're walking around or feel a rush of blood when you stand up. This is normal and is due to the shape of the vagina; the blood pools inside you whilst you're sitting down and finds its way out when you stand up. Many women also find they bleed more when they breastfeed or express milk, as the hormones involved in breastfeeding cause their uterus to contract.

As days go by, the bleeding should become lighter in colour. The second phase of the lochia is pinkish-brown and will last until two or three weeks postpartum, while the last phase can last until six weeks or more but should be whitish-yellow in colour, so it's less of a nuisance.

Managing the bleeding

Giant cotton knickers are a good bet for the first week or two, especially if you've had a caesarean and your normal pants sit around the scar line. Women who've had caesareans often recommend disposable knickers because they are very soft and don't irritate the scar. You can also get padded 'hospital knickers' that offer extra cushioning and hold pads in place.

Stock up on thick pads. Midwives advise that the large, plain cotton maternity pads they give out in hospitals are better for preventing infections than the modern, low-profile, ultra-absorbent pads that you buy for your period. This makes sense as the latter are generally covered in two layers of plastic, with another layer of plastic on the back, whereas cotton allows the area to breathe.

Just remember that your body is open and raw during the first few weeks after giving birth. You're more vulnerable than

Tip: Sit on a lily pad

Sarah found wearing pads so uncomfortable that she preferred to sit on a disposable incontinence sheet for the first week or two, covering her lap with a blanket, to give her vagina more airflow and freedom. She accepts that bleeding out onto a lily pad is not everyone's cup of tea, but it worked for her, because having a pad in her underwear rubbed her graze and stuck to the healing tissue. She entertained many a visitor like this, sitting on her absorbent bed pad, and those she didn't mention it to were none the wiser. (A disposable sheet like this might also be useful overnight when you're breastfeeding to reduce the number of times you need to change your bed sheets, to catch those unanticipated newborn wees, or as a portable nappy mat.)

usual to infection spreading up from your vagina, so avoid tampons, swimming in public pools and having sex whilst you're experiencing discharge. Wash with water, change your pads regularly, wear clean cotton pants and try a healing sitz bath (see page 80) if you feel like it.

When to call a doctor

If your bleeding doesn't follow the guide given above, and you feel worried about it, don't hesitate to get some professional medical advice. Here are a few important indicators to look out for when things aren't quite right.

Increase in blood loss – If at any point your blood loss starts to increase, you could have a postpartum haemorrhage and should contact your midwife or doctor. This is more common after a C-section but can also occur after a vaginal birth. Most postpartum haemorrhages occur within 24 hours of birth, but they can happen anything up to 12 weeks later. As well as uncontrolled bleeding, symptoms include shivering and feeling clammy, nausea, weakness, dizziness, an increased heart rate and drop in blood pressure. If your bleeding is very heavy and any of these occur, contact the emergency services immediately.

Bright red blood after a week – The blood loss should become increasingly less red, and should not go back to being red having become lighter in colour. If it does suddenly appear brighter red in colour, this is another sign of a haemorrhage.

Extra-large clots – Small and even large clots are normal, but you should contact a doctor immediately about any clot that is extra-large – bigger than a golf ball or a plum.

Bad smell – It's possible that bad-smelling lochia is the only symptom you'll have of an infection, so it's important that you pay attention to the odour. Other symptoms of infection include a fever, chills, pain in the lower abdomen and ongoing cramping.

Sitz baths

Born in 1799, the Austrian Vincenz Priessnitz, founder of modern hydrotherapy, believed water could cure anything from insanity to poisoning. He treated kings and queens with water therapies at his village clinic in the former Austrian Silesia (now the Czech Republic). Among the therapies he developed was the sitz bath, and it remains one of the oldest and most important hydrotherapy procedures around.

For a few pounds, you can buy a sort of potty that goes over the loo, which you fill with water and sit on. Or you can sit in a bath. When it comes to what to fill it with, there are different schools of thought: you can use either hot or cold water, and you can choose to add salts, herbs and essential oils – or not. No one really knows what works best. Using cold water makes sense, because we know that cold reduces inflammation by decreasing blood flow. A 1986 study suggests that a cold sitz bath is best for pain relief, and more recent studies suggest that cold helps reduce inflammation. Heat, however, increases blood flow, and blood contains nutrients and oxygen that enable healing. For this reason, other proponents of sitz baths – including traditional Chinese medicine practitioners – recommend you sit in hot water to promote blood flow. In short, if it makes you feel better, it doesn't matter which you choose.

There is also limited research on the effect of adding salts or witch hazel to the water – both of which reportedly speed up healing. In Iran, doctors recommend aromatherapy – essential oils taken from the roots, leaves, seeds or flowers of plants – and another study suggests that both olive oil and a few drops of lavender essential oil in a warm bath might speed up healing.

In the UK, the official line is that, whilst things like Epsom salts can feel soothing for some, they don't make a difference to the healing when compared with plain water. If the scent of lavender will make you feel better, go for it.

There are any number of herbal mixtures, tea bags, essential oils and healing salts on the market. Just avoid using salt if you've had stitches, as it can dissolve them too quickly.

Uterine contractions

In the first days of breastfeeding, I was gripped by pleasure-pain. The baby's suckling at my breast was not unpleasant, but the oxytocin it stimulated caused my uterus, which had once housed the baby, to cramp as it returned to something like its original size. The accompanying pain was a welcome indication of the fact that I was shrinking. (Not all women feel the cramping the first time round – with subsequent babies it's common to feel it more clearly.) And the cramping explains why, in the early days, breastfeeding stimulates blood loss.

The uterus (or womb) is mostly muscle, and pregnancy stretches it. In the first few days after you give birth it weighs around a kilogram and, immediately after expelling the placenta, it is still the size of a grapefruit and reaches almost up to your belly button. It then starts to contract and will drop down by about a finger's breadth every day. Painkillers can help ease the discomfort of this, as can gentle massage. And while breastfeeding helps the uterus to shrink, there is no clear evidence to say that the muscle contracts more slowly in women who don't breastfeed or who have C-sections.

A midwife should check the progress of your uterus by pressing gently on your tummy when she sees you. It should feel firm like a grapefruit for the first few days after birth and contract by about a centimetre a day. By two weeks postpartum it should have settled back down into your pelvis. By six weeks, it should have completed its journey, returning to a weight of around 60 to 80 grams (from approximately a kilo), just slightly more than the womb of a woman who's never given birth.

Cervix

This short cylinder of muscle that connects the vagina to the womb was your baby's gateway into the world. I'd never considered my own cervix until I hit my due date, at which point it became an obsession. The midwife kept telling me, in very specific terms, what it needed to do: to tilt, thin, shorten, soften and open. This was too much for me, so I focused instead on the image of the baby's head wearing away at a spongy wall until it gave way.

When nothing had happened and I was a week overdue, I decided that my cervix was a wilful and unhelpful body part, and that no amount of ungainly sex, pineapples, long walks, scrubbing floors or raspberry leaf tea (each of which is reputed to help induce labour, and each of which I self-medicated with on a daily basis) could influence it. Eventually, ten days late, it did all of the things it was meant to do, without intervention, and admiration replaced my frustrations.

The cervix is usually about 4 to 5 centimetres long, but after childbirth it hangs down into the vagina, swollen, bruised and dilated. (Rarely, in just 0.2 per cent of cases, it can also be torn or cut.) In the course of the first 12 to 18 hours after birth, your body produces special cells to rehabilitate it, shorten it and firm it up. By 30 hours after birth, your cervix should be around 5 to 6 centimetres long, and six months afterwards it will be around 2.9 centimetres, just slightly longer than before. Within two or three days, the aperture that opened up will be just 2 or 3 centimetres across, and a week afterwards it'll just be 1 centimetre. By four weeks, it should be closed, but not necessarily fully healed.

7

Breasts and Breastfeeding

My mum has a picture at home, a watercolour that once belonged to her mother, of a woman nursing an infant. The woman, in her gold frame and wearing a pale blue shawl, looks so serene. My mum used to gaze at it during the long nights of sitting up and breastfeeding me and my sister. I used to gaze at that picture, too, and I later imagined myself as a mother, captured in such a moment of serenity.

I remain fond of the picture, but I also blame it for my false hopes. While it can be the most intimate and spellbindingly beautiful thing imaginable, breastfeeding can also be painful, messy and stressful – and that's if it works. Sometimes it does not, and with the pressure we put on women to breastfeed in the UK, this can feel devastating.

I was very lucky to have more than enough milk, but that still didn't mean it was easy. On day three, when my milk came in, Philip and I did little but marvel (him) and express horror (me) at my boobs. They were enormous and alarmingly pressurised. When the milk flowed it was a tsunami that permeated everything. I covered whatever I touched in breastmilk – my clothes, the baby's clothes, Philip's clothes and our house. Breastmilk is so revered in our culture but so unpleasant when soured on your sofa. The laundry piled up, keeping my husband chained to the machine, and my enormous breasts went on producing. At times, it felt like I was choking our little bean with the pressure of a fire hose.

When the baby and I did manage to sit and feed in harmony, I always seemed to be without something – my book, my phone, water (always water) or a cushion to support my back. As a result, I was constantly reliant on Philip. If I was left alone, once the baby had latched on and was feeding correctly, I would endure anything – boredom, thirst or pain – in order to not move. Some women do find breastfeeding easy – one friend describes how she and her first baby 'just clicked' – but many do not. Once you get the hang of it, however, it is incredibly rewarding and convenient, while providing the best possible nutrients and ultimate source of comfort for your child.

If you don't find it easy and want help, La Leche League provides amazing free resources; a global organisation, they're like the Samaritans of breastfeeding mothers. I was once losing my mind having spent six hours trying to feed the baby and stumbled across the number of their national helpline.

'Hello?' one of their volunteers, a grandmotherly Australian woman, answered. It seemed I had been diverted to her landline.

I told her that my breasts fired like water cannon and that my son refused to feed from them. It was 1 p.m. and he hadn't drunk anything all day. Voice cracking, I started to cry.

Leslie, as she was called, gently explained the problem of oversupply, something I'd never heard of before, reassured me that my baby wasn't going to starve, and told me how to manage things. My guardian angel of breastmilk and sanity, she had come out of nowhere and, within about ten minutes, talked me down from being a stressy milk pusher (who, if I were my baby, I wouldn't want to feed from either) into the calm, relaxed mother I'd been before. Not only that, I had a plan – and it worked.

The message here is simple: if you're struggling, don't do it alone. Reach out to someone, anyone, whether it's a friend, family member or your very own Leslie, because you never know who might be able to help.

> *Lucia, GP and mother of three:*
> *'I think it's one of the hardest things you can do, to take on responsibility for another human being. It's huge. I thought that I was going to be well prepared for being a mother because I'd done sleep deprivation; as a junior doctor, I'd spent whole weekends with no sleep looking after my 60-odd patients on the wards. But actually nothing could have prepared me for how I was going to feel once I'd had a baby for three or four weeks that was breastfeeding every two hours, 24 hours a day. And because I was breastfeeding, I didn't seem to be able to hand her to anyone else. I think there is real pressure not to admit it if you're not coping, but actually it is fine to say, I'm not coping, this is really hard.'*

'Breast is best'

When a friend struggled to breastfeed her son, I harboured secret envy, eyeing up her neat bottles and fresh-smelling clothes. Another friend who lives in France simply chose not to breastfeed for more than a few months. I'd somehow been inculcated with the urge to breastfeed from a young age, and never thought to question it. My friend in France, however, had an instinct that she wouldn't particularly like it, and she was right; she didn't. Instead, she fed the baby for two or three months then gave it infant probiotics alongside formula, and everyone was happy with the outcome.

Many cultures, mine included, put great weight on the importance of breastfeeding, and understandably so. It is magical if you can do it – for the baby's immune system, for your ability to soothe them, for the ease of not having to bother with sterilising bottles, for reducing the risk of scary prospects like childhood leukemia and Sudden Infant Death Syndrome, and even for your child's brain development and your own health. Plus, you can still enjoy a glass of wine when you're breastfeeding – experts say that if you're sober enough to look after a baby responsibly, you're sober enough to breastfeed, and the amount in your milk will never exceed that in your bloodstream.

On the other hand, evidence also suggests that it's not such a big deal if you don't or can't breastfeed. France has the lowest breastfeeding rates in the Western world – of the 70 per cent of mothers who start breastfeeding, those who do so exclusively do it for only seven weeks on average. French feminists argue that, in romanticising motherhood with 'natural birth' and encouraging breastfeeding for months on end, we are imposing a regression on ourselves by making our lives harder. In France, if you do insist on breastfeeding, you may well be told by your doctor after four to eight weeks that you've hit *l'étape biberon* – the bottle stage – when your baby needs more milk than you have. Despite this, life expectancy in France is higher than it is in the UK, and under-five mortality rates are the same. Basically, if breastfeeding doesn't work out for you, remember the French approach: a bottle beats an unhappy mama, hands down.

Mariana had an emergency caesarean and breastfed her baby for three days before noticing something was wrong:

'My boobs were huge and rock-hard, I had milk, but something was not adding up. Newborns don't eat that much, but no matter what I did his hunger was not going away. My hormones were all over the place and I started panicking, crying – what's wrong with me? The midwife said, shall we give him a bit of a bottle and see if that helps? As soon as they gave him some bottle he stopped crying and went to sleep. Oh shit, I thought, something is not working. I had a breast augmentation when I was younger. Could that have something to do with it?

'I bought a massive breastfeeding pillow, hired a lactation consultant, got fenugreek pills and kept feeding for a whole week – but I was exhausted by the end because he was not sleeping more than 30 to 40 minutes. Everything was so painful, he'd eroded my nipple down to half and it was bleeding like an open wound. The lactation consultant said you can also express with a pump to get your supply up. So then I was breastfeeding, and pumping whenever I wasn't – but his weight still dropped to a point where it was almost scary.

'I gave it two more weeks of manically trying to breastfeed and pump, but at that point I was losing it. My mum could see that I was falling apart. The breastfeeding consultant was saying, you have to keep going, be strong. My mum was like, fuck this. We're going to buy some bottles and some formula. I stopped breastfeeding because my nipples were so raw, but I was still expressing every two hours, waking up to pump even when he was sleeping. After two months, I stopped. I have a history of mental health problems and my mum and husband were so concerned that they pushed me to give up. I *felt a massive failure for not doing the job I was meant to as a mother, but after a few months, I thought – well, I can make myself miserable, or I can get over it.*

'I have heard of a lot of people being pressured into breast-feeding. I did get a lot of "you should try, and you should keep trying, because it's worth it". The lactation consultant was a bit militant, but the midwives were not as pushy as I expected. In the end, I think the worst pressure came from me. It was hard for me to enjoy being a mother for the first few months because I was so stressed and sad and guilty. I don't want that to happen again if I can help it, especially if there's an alternative that is absolutely safe and suitable. My son turned out pretty fine, after all.'

Formula feeding from the start

Women who make an informed decision not to breastfeed (or to stop early) do so for a variety of very personal reasons, from practical concerns to past sexual experiences, and should not be judged or asked to defend their choice. Constantly being asked how you're feeding your child, however, might make you feel uncomfortable or defensive. You might like to decide on a line that makes you feel confident – 'I'd have liked to breastfeed but it didn't work for us', for example – and if you don't want to have to explain your choices, move the discussion on. Once you've made your decision not to breastfeed, no doctor, midwife or nurse should pressure you into changing your mind. And you're not obliged to share your reasoning with anyone unless you want to.

If you do opt out of breastfeeding from the outset, you'll likely still have to grapple with a bit of milk while your body adjusts. While you were pregnant, the placenta was producing high levels of oestrogen and progesterone, which inhibited the production of breastmilk. When these hormone levels crash, the body goes into milk-producing mode, spurred on by the hormone prolactin. If you then don't feed or express at all, your body will start to counterbalance the effects of pro-lactin with another hormone to halt the production line. It should take between a week and ten days for the milk to stop. During this time, your breasts might feel uncomfortable, so see the advice for engorgement; massage often, apply ice or frozen peas, and take ibuprofen for soreness. Express for comfort only if you need to – for example, if the pain is too much, or if you get any tender lumps (see page 99 for advice on blocked ducts and mastitis). There is, unfortunately, as of yet no magic bullet to dry up milk supply. Despite popular belief, there is little good evidence to show that consuming sage or applying cabbage leaves will reduce your supply, and only limited evidence to suggest that pseudoephedrine – a decongestant commonly known as Sudafed – works (and it's not licensed for this purpose). Don't bind your breasts or restrict your fluid intake, either – neither is shown to help, and you may do more harm than good.

Engorgement

Engorgement is most likely to be a problem around the time that your milk first comes in. Breasts feel painful, firm and very full and, if they stay engorged for too long, your chances of developing mastitis or blocked ducts increase (see page 99), so feed often to get the milk moving.

There is evidence to show that massage helps. Try massaging your breasts in the shower or bath under warm water, with strokes that go towards the nipple. Doctors and midwives also recommend you apply heat to the breasts before feeding, then put something cold on them afterwards. Studies show that this can help with both the pain and inflammation. For the cold compress, you can wet a breast pad and put it in the freezer so it's ice-cold. To be clever, you can freeze it on the base of an upturned bowl so it comes out breast-shaped and fits flush to you. For heat, you can use a flannel soaked in hot water (which cools down a bit too quickly) or a sock containing rice that's been heated up for a minute in the microwave. If it gets really painful, try expressing – you need to keep the milk moving to prevent blockages and infection.

Some women find that putting raw chilled or frozen cabbage leaves inside their bra helps. There is some science behind this. Cabbages contain glucosinolates, which convert to a substance known as mustard oil, a traditional remedy for inflammation (as well as joint pain). Before you run to the fridge, though, there isn't enough evidence for official medical guidelines to support cabbage leaves for engorgement. However, numerous studies do suggest that chilled cabbage leaves are just as good as hot and cold compresses when it comes to reducing inflammation. Cheap and easy, the only potential downside is that cabbage leaves may reduce milk supply over time (although, again, there is no good evidence for this).

The let-down

When your body gets the urge to feed your baby, it cues the let-down reflex. Two hormones are responsible for this: prolactin and oxytocin. This sensation varies hugely. For one friend it felt like sweat prickling her brow, but for another it was like barbed wire being pulled through her nipple. I experienced more of a burning sensation. However painful it is for you, the let-down doesn't last long, so if you have persistent pain then it's likely to be caused by something else.

In some women, the reflex initiates a fast rush of milk that may overwhelm your baby. Mine came out like a pressure-washer at first, with up to eight individual jets at a time. I learned to catch it, with a towel, a cup or a hand-pump, taking the worst off until it settled into a trickle, but within a few months my baby had learnt to handle the high-pressure flow.

If you're pumping, you'll learn what works for you to get the milk going. A lot of women hold their baby, look at a picture of them, or imagine them suckling. Milk comes into both boobs at once, so it's common to leak from the one you're not feeding with, particularly at the start. For this reason, if you're expressing, pumping on both sides at once can speed things up as well as boost production. To catch the milk from the other boob, you can use breast pads – either reusable ones or disposable ones (which are more absorbent but more expensive over time and less kind to the environment). Or you can get a small, reusable device known as a breast shell to collect milk from the spare breast whilst you feed on the other.

Unfortunately, the let-down reflex is not perfect and you may find your breasts suddenly wanting to feed someone who is not your baby, such as characters on television, strangers who are kind to you in train stations, or your partner. I've heard the let-down described as our equivalent of an erection – an involuntary response that sends fluid rushing to fulfil a task inside you, full of enthusiasm but occasionally misdirected. Again, breast pads are your friend.

If you find breastfeeding a bit fraught to start with, it's worth knowing that it won't always be this way. You will soon know what you're doing, your milk will settle down, and at some point you'll become the serene woman in my mum's picture.

> *Laura recalls the embarrassing consequences of her powerful let-down reflex:*
> 'I was sitting in a café about to feed my baby. My let-down was super strong at the time, and I was just getting the baby into position when I heard someone call my name. I jerked my head up and there was my ex-boyfriend, who I hadn't seen for years, standing at the table. My milk squirted up at him and I got him in the eye.'

Switching sides

The less full your breast is, the higher the fat content of the milk. For this reason, you shouldn't switch boobs just for the sake of it as soon as the first boob feels less full. The National Childbirth Trust (NCT) says that, because each mother–baby feeding pair is different, there is no one-size-fits-all approach, so rather than watch the clock, you should pay attention to your baby. The NCT recommends that you switch only when it seems your baby has had enough from one breast; they might show this by coming off it, or by slowing their feeding right down. Not all babies drink from both breasts during a feed; some will just want one, while others will want to switch sides multiple times.

Nipples and breast pain

You have just two highly sensitive nubbins of flesh to sustain a human being the size of a lapdog for months, so you need

Nursing bras

While you might not wear your nursing bra for terribly long, it is worth investing in a good one, because a badly fitting bra can obstruct your milk and lead to blocked ducts and mastitis. If you have bigger breasts, you can get bras with soft underwires, which are fine as long as they fit really well and don't pinch or squeeze. Whatever bra you choose, make sure it is comfortable. Go to a shop and get fitted if in any doubt.

to look after them. During pregnancy, your nipples can hurt because of hormonal changes. After birth, however, pain can be a warning sign that something is wrong. Some women do feel pain during breastfeeding for no good reason – they just seem to experience it that way. But often a shallow latch, tongue tie, large nipples or even just a tricky start that took its toll on the nipples is to blame. And once you start, you can't take a break for recovery else your milk will dry up; the feeding needs to be constant.

Pain is one of the top reasons why women stop breast-feeding early, but take heart from the fact that most women find it goes away within seven to ten days postpartum. If it is painful and your nipples are raw, ask your midwife to check your latch, or look up the NHS guidance online. Also, check your baby's mouth for signs of oral thrush, which can infect your nipples; it can look a bit like cottage cheese on the tongue that can't be wiped off easily, or white spots around the mouth. If you do get nipple thrush, it's likely to result in severe pain for up to an hour in both breasts or nipples after each feed. There is no need to stop breastfeeding – your GP will prescribe a gel or ointment to treat you and the baby together. Many women also develop back, neck or shoulder pain due to the way they sit whilst breastfeeding. (See Chapter 17 on musculoskeletal pain for more on this.)

> *Zara experienced pain throughout her first few months of breastfeeding, and believes it was not because she (or the baby) was doing something wrong:*
> 'I found breastfeeding incredibly painful. The breastfeeding groups say that if it hurts then you're doing it wrong. I think that's really unhelpful. I had my latch checked, I had everything checked by a lactation specialist, and there was nothing wrong. The baby was thriving on it and loved his boobie, but still it was painful for me for the first three months. I had to bite down on something to get through it. My sister had exactly the same issue. So I just don't think that sweeping statement, that you're doing it wrong if it's hurting, is fair.'

Cracks and soreness

Between 80 and 90 per cent of breastfeeding women experience nipples that are sore (when the skin is intact) and cracked (when it's wounded and broken). This can be down to anything from the baby's position (see above – check your latch) or using soap that's dried them out. It can be excruciating and feel like the baby has taken a chunk out of you. Keep feeding on the painful nipple, but feed from the least-painful nipple first, as the beginning of the feed will involve the most suction. You can also take paracetamol or ibuprofen at least half an hour before, and try applying an ice pack to the nipple before feeding to anaesthetise it.

If your skin is sore but not broken, pause before reaching for a treatment pad or ointment. A 2019 review of scientific literature by the UK's Breastfeeding Network concluded that there is no evidence that anything helps. You should save the ointments for when the skin is broken because sore nipples alone don't need it; check your positioning instead. There is, as with so many postnatal health problems, little research on the subject, but experts caution that applying products to unbroken skin may actually contribute to the problem by making cracks more likely.

If the skin is already broken, there are two approaches to healing: keeping the nipples moist, or allowing them to dry out. Since the 1960s, scientists have known that wounds heal faster when they're kept moist rather than dry, which is why women are often advised to apply breast milk, lanolin or Vaseline to the nipples. By keeping the wound moist you also reduce pain and prevent scabs that the baby could pull off when feeding, thus undoing all of your body's hard work.

A 2014 review of evidence, however, found that applying nothing or breast milk can be as good as, if not better than, expensive ointments such as lanolin (sold as the brand Lansinoh). Breastmilk is thought to have healing properties, while the Breastfeeding Network advises that Vaseline, which is cheaper and less allergenic, or purified lanolin can help. Vaseline (petroleum jelly) is a petrol by-product and is often slammed by environmentalists and proponents of natural beauty, but it's been trusted to moisturise the lips of babies in special care units for generations thanks to its ability to lock in moisture and its absence of allergens. Hydrogel pads are becoming popular but evidence shows they can be linked to higher rates of infection. And some women report success with silver nipple cups, which follow the principle of moist healing. You line the cups with breastmilk then place them over the nipples after feeding, to prevent friction and stop the wounds drying out. In 2015, a group of Italian women with cracked nipples used either silver cups or standard healing methods. After two days there was no difference, but by seven days those with silver cups had healed quicker. Whatever treatment you choose, patience is the key, as is correcting your positioning and the baby's latch. Lots of women consider pumping to give the nipple a break but experts caution that this involves more suction than breastfeeding, which only exerts negative pressure on the nipple at the start. Try changing your breastfeeding position instead to one that feels more comfortable.

Annabel resorted to Madonna-esque breast shells to dry out the wounds on her nipples:
'The baby had literally taken out a part of my nipple. It was so bad, my wound kept bleeding and bleeding. I was pumping, putting on lanolin cream, and changing my pads every hour. It was never going to heal unless I let it clot and scab so I bought these weird nipple domes – Medela breast shells – that you wear in your bra to keep the wound away from any contact and allow it to heal in the air. They are almost Madonna-esque, with openings for the areola. I could also have walked around topless for two weeks but it just wasn't practical. Instead, I looked like Barberella – but it worked!'

Blocked ducts

Your ducts act like highways to transport the milk from inside the breast to the nipple, and the milk needs to be able to flow freely – otherwise it can get clogged. With a blocked duct, you'll usually have a hard lump or area of engorgement near to the blockage that is tender, swollen, hot and red, although it's possible that you just have an area that's sore without the lump. After feeding, it will feel less painful and the lump should have gone down. It might be painful to feed or pump from the affected breast, especially during the let-down, but it's important that you do so in order to clear it.

Feeding your baby frequently and thoroughly is the most effective treatment for blocked ducts (and mastitis).

Take painkillers, start each feed on the painful breast for the next 12 hours and make sure you empty it fully (feeding your baby from the boob with the blocked duct is more effective than pumping). Massage towards the nipple in between feeds, and apply heat to the area before a feed (see page 92 for tips on making heat packs). Try running a wide-toothed comb or anything firm along the breast towards the nipple to try to draw out the blockage (this works especially well in the shower) and massage in the direction of the nipple whilst the baby feeds. You can even try feeding the baby while leaning over it – known as 'dangle feeding' – as it's believed that gravity can help dislodge the blockage.

Early mastitis

A few weeks after my son's birth, I woke up in the night feeling shivery and with an intense pain in my left boob. The next morning, I noticed that a triangular wedge of breast tissue looked bright red and angry. By now, alarm bells were ringing; mastitis was kicking in. I massaged and pumped and fed and showered in hot water on repeat all day. The next night it was neither better nor worse. After two days of this, I finally started to feel some relief.

If you act swiftly at the first sign of an infection, it's possible to catch it early before it develops into full-blown mastitis. Firstly, lactation specialists advise you take 400 milligrams of ibuprofen every eight hours to reduce the swelling (or paracetamol, if you can't take ibuprofen). And take paracetamol concurrently if you need to for pain relief. Otherwise, do the same as you would for blocked ducts but also apply ice after feeds (or try putting a chilled cabbage leaf in your bra, see page 92), and massage as much as you can. Swimming – in particular front crawl and backstroke where you're circling your arms around – is said to help, or any exercise where you're swinging your arms about to get things moving. If it doesn't start improving within 24 hours, you may need antibiotics.

Mastitis

Anyone who's had mastitis may well break into expletives if you ask them what it was like. Imagine your breasts being stuffed with burning coals while your nipples express razor blades. Also known as 'boob flu', that is how mastitis was once described to me. It can happen to anyone but is most common in the first three months after birth. It is essentially an inflammatory response, which sounds manageable, but it is excruciating and can knock you down like the flu. It usually comes on quickly and, like a blocked duct, affects just one breast at a time. The symptoms are largely the same as for a blocked duct and early mastitis but far more intense and all-encompassing, and you'll need to contact your health visitor or GP for help.

You'll likely have a temperature of 38.5°C or more and a large area of the breast will feel hot and painful to touch. There might be one particularly red and swollen area, and, as with a blocked duct, you might have a lump or hard patch, or the whole breast may even be red and inflamed. You may have nipple discharge, which can be white or blood-stained, and flu-like symptoms. The pain, which can feel like a burning sensation, is also more intense and can be constant or come on when you're feeding. All this in a highly sensitive erogenous zone: it's no wonder you hear new mums saying they never want anyone – partners included – to touch their boobs ever again.

Treatment includes everything you'd do for a blocked duct and early mastitis, but also antibiotics. You can continue to feed your baby whilst you're taking antibiotics, but be aware that your baby might have some diarrhoea or be a bit colicky for a few days, and look out for signs of thrush in yourself and your baby due to the antibiotics. If you can't feed your baby from the affected boob, use a pump to drain it; it's vital that you empty it regularly and thoroughly. Try to get some help with the baby and stay in bed if you can. Keep hydrated and eat well to support your immune system.

Mira struggled first with blocked ducts, then mastitis:
'People think mastitis is just a sore boob. It's not – it completely takes over your whole body. I don't think I've ever been so ill. And you've got this tiny baby who's totally reliant on you so you can't just have a day in bed. I had a full-on fever and boobs that were bursting, painful, red-hot; it was excruciating to feed him. I had antibiotics but there

isn't much else you can do. I tried all the home remedies – hot compresses, cold compresses, getting the baby to feed. In the end the baby developed an aversion to feeding on the poorly boob so I used to squeeze the milk out while lying on my front in the bath. Someone told me that the best thing was to get someone with a forceful suck to suck out the gunk. I mentioned this to my partner; he refused point blank. Then I got a text from my mum offering to do it. I contemplated what it'd be like, having to look down and see my mum sucking at my tits. How would I look her in the eye afterwards? I did actually stop to consider it because it was that bad.'

Supply issues

Boobs make milk on a supply-and-demand basis: the more your baby feeds (particularly during the evenings and the first half of the night, which is when things reset), the more your boobs will make. This is a book in itself, but remember that breasts that feel empty usually still give milk, that babies feed for comfort as well as food, every baby is different, and your breasts adjust.

Not enough milk: To increase your milk production, experts advise you feed as often as possible, try to switch breasts two or three times during each feed, keep up the night feeds, ditch the dummy, and try compressing the breasts to keep the baby feeding by boosting the flow. Even if it may look like the baby isn't getting milk towards the end of a feed, it is probably just taking in the richer hind milk, which it swallows more slowly. Taking fenugreek, a herb typically used in Indian cooking, may also help boost your supply; evidence suggests it could be more effective in the first few days post-partum than after two weeks.

Too much milk: You have two things to think about: managing your supply issues in the longer-term, and managing your and your baby's feeding experience in the shorter term. In terms of your supply, experts say you shouldn't try to reduce it in the first month because it needs to find its own rhythm, but after that you could – ideally with guidance – try reducing it by feeding on one breast for a number of hours at a time before switching to the next. In the short term, you can release excess pressure by massaging your boobs, let-down into a tea towel or cup if yours is particularly forceful, and express a little milk as you need to – in between feeds for comfort, or before feeds to make it easier for your baby and to ensure they don't get too much of the low-fat, high-sugar fore milk. You can also try lying back with the baby on top to reduce the flow, and help them to latch onto a full breast by pinching the skin around the nipple. In my case, no matter what I did my boobs continued to produce too much milk until my baby stopped feeding at night, at which point my supply quickly settled down. (For more, see the Resources section for an article published by the Breastfeeding Basics website on oversupply.)

Dysphoric milk ejection reflex

In 2007, an American lactation consultant called Alia Mac-rina Heise gave birth to her third child at home. It was a perfect birth and she felt relaxed in the weeks that fol-lowed, with plenty of support, but she couldn't shake the instinct that something was not right. She experienced 'a sickening hollow feeling in the pit of my stomach', combined with intense feelings of worthlessness and shame, and even fleeting moments of being suicidal. She decided it was probably the 'baby blues' or postnatal depression, but somehow that didn't feel right. She had no history of depression and, when she analysed the feelings of guilt or worthlessness, she realised there was nothing behind them – they were just random emotions without substance. The negative feelings only lasted for one or two minutes before disappearing, but they were so overwhelming that she had to concentrate on getting through them as she would a contraction. The rest of the time, she felt fine.

One day, browsing an internet forum, she came across a thread called 'Only When Nursing'. In it, she read about dozens of other women who were experiencing the same thing, who had linked it to breastfeeding. At that point, she realised that her feelings weren't linked to nursing per se but to the let-down reflex. She had a lot of milk and her breasts would release it whenever they got full throughout the day; the negative emotions would overwhelm her just before the let-down. It was a revelation.

Over a decade later, Alia is now in demand as a speaker at breastfeeding and midwifery forums, having coined the term Dysphoric Milk Ejection Reflex (D-MER) to describe a condition experienced by women the world over. Some mothers describe it as if Dementors, those most-feared mythical creatures of J.K. Rowling's imaginings, were sucking their soul out for a minute or so whenever they started feeding. Alia believes the condition is linked to the fall in dopamine levels that helps to trigger the milk ejection reflex.

The condition is often misdiagnosed as postnatal depression or anxiety, Alia says. Whilst there is currently no treatment, Alia has found that most mothers are just relieved to hear an explanation for their feelings, which helps them cope with it.

About two months after my baby was born, I was lucky to experience the opposite feeling: when I started a feed, I would often experience a short period of euphoria around the time of the let-down. Each time it happened, it reminded me of dancing to trance music in the early noughties, and I would revel in the irony of this.

Insufficient glandular tissue

The size of your boobs has nothing to do with how much milk you make; it's fat that gives you big boobs, glandular tissue that makes milk. Roughly one in 20 women, however, have insufficient glandular tissue, which can cause milk supply issues – but the condition is persistently missed by lactation consultants and midwives. A Washington academic and breastfeeding consultant, Diana Cassar-Uhl, has written a book about it called *Finding Sufficiency*, and believes it's linked to diet, insulin resistance and a woman's BMI – particularly during childhood, when her breast tissue was developing.

Indicators of insufficient glandular tissue include having a flat space between your boobs of more than four centimetres, one breast significantly larger than the other, breasts that are narrow at the base and long rather than round, and having bigger areolae than you might expect. And, if your boobs don't change during or after pregnancy, it may be that you'll have supply issues. To help, you can try a supplement or drug to increase your supply, such as fenugreek or domperidone, top up with formula or donated milk and use a breastfeeding supplementer – a tube that still allows the baby to suckle at the breast while drinking formula or expressed milk at the same time. You can also just have your baby suckle at the breast, even if your supply isn't sustaining them.

Rhiannon never made sufficient milk for her baby – but that didn't stop her breastfeeding:

'I was pumping 15 times a day but she was getting all the milk she needed through formula alone. "Oh, it'll all be fine, you're anxious, you had a caesarean," the midwives said. I went on domperidone, goat's rue, everything there was. But if I didn't feed her for 12 hours, there was no change in the texture of my breasts. Only afterwards it became clear to me that I had insufficient glandular tissue, linked to my nutrition. If you're overweight during adolescence, your breast tissue doesn't always develop properly; the classic effect is like a snooker ball in a sock. Despite that, we had a breastfeeding relationship for about 22 months, because there's more to it than just milk. There would be drops of milk – at the most – but she craved the comfort. You often get a lot of frowns when women decide to mix feed; we should try to be more sensitive of the fact that, for lots of reasons, exclusive breast-feeding doesn't always work, and that mixed feeding is OK. Instead, the education focuses on the fact that every woman can breastfeed if they try hard enough; that's not true. I never felt any true support when I was going through it – just an eye-roll, "you're just a middle-class mum being neurotic," and the silent assumption that I just didn't want to breastfeed. That couldn't have been further from the truth.'

Hydration

Expect to be very, very thirsty while breastfeeding. The poet Hollie McNish tells a devastating story about this in a poem called 'Water Bottles', written when her daughter was one week old. On the first night, her partner Dee put a cup of water on the table next to Hollie, who was feeding her daughter on the sofa, before going to bed. He woke to find Hollie and the baby sitting at the other end of the sofa, Hollie gazing desperately at the water. Later that night, the baby finally fell asleep, but once more Hollie found herself sitting in the wrong place to reach her water. She wept with thirst and exasperation. The next night, her partner put out four cups of water, so that she always had access to one. Hollie brought a cup gratefully to her lips, but the baby kicked it over just before she could drink from it and she sat in the dark with a wet crotch for three hours, crying again. On the last night, her partner put bottles of water with lids on every surface of the house. This time the water didn't spill, but still she cried, *while whispering to her baby, 'I'm not very good at this.'*

So, cover the house in spill-proof bottles, cry when you feel like it, and eat well (see Chapter 9).

8

Rest and Sleep

The UK's first maternity hospital, which opened in 1767, was called the General Lying-In Hospital, named after the month-long period of bed-rest that doctors routinely prescribed to women after giving birth. The tradition of staying in bed after birth persisted for another 200 years. If you gave birth in the 1970s, you'd expect to stay in hospital for at least ten days afterwards, and the baby would go to a nursery at night to ensure you were well rested before going home. In the early eighties, it was still a week.

Given the state of our hospitals today, I'm not sure anyone would welcome spending such a long time on a postnatal ward unnecessarily, but in choosing to recover at home many of us have lost our respect for this important period of healing and recovery. (Although, interestingly, the government's MAT B1 forms, which you fill in to qualify for maternity pay, still refer not to the birth but to 'the confinement'.)

While Western societies have lost the practice of lying-in (bed-rest and recuperation) in favour of trying to 'bounce back', women still practise a version of it all over the world – and, wherever you go, from the Amazon to the Far East, the hallmark rituals of recovery are curiously similar. They recognise that a new mother has just experienced a major medical event and is severely depleted. She needs bed-rest and privacy, while relatives keep her warm, comfortable and well-nourished, with healing foods (see Chapter 9) and massage. In China, *zuo you zi*, or 'sitting the month', lasts for a lunar cycle and dictates that you do nothing – brush your hair, carry your child or leave the house – so that your body can recalibrate. In Malawi, the new mum gets her own bed for a month, next to her husband's. These practices have existed for millennia and are believed to help with recovery in the long term. I discovered all of this too late, over a year after giving birth, by which point I still didn't feel fully recovered – and no wonder; I'd dragged my poor body out to the pub for lunch on day three.

Proponents of the month-long rest period say it helps prevent problems later in life, as staying in bed takes the downward pressure off your organs, privates and pelvic floor as they recover from birth. But scientists are not sure that literally lying in bed for a month is such a good thing. Studies show that limiting physical activity is bad for muscles and cardiovascular health and makes postpartum depression (see page 131) more likely. One study found that, while a period of rest actually helped some women get back to their pre-baby weight, it left them feeling sad and raised their glucose and cholesterol levels.

How much you do in the weeks after the birth is your choice – but don't be a busy fool. Allow yourself to be looked after, nourish and protect your body, and get as much sleep and rest as possible. As Ross J. Barr, a London acupuncturist specialising in women's health, says to clients again and again, 'The best way to take care of your baby is to make sure you're in good condition. Because if you're not, it affects your baby – so you really have to put yourself first.'

Personally, rather than feel guilty about getting it wrong

the first time (guilt being the other thing women are pre-programmed for), I will try to do it differently next time: to rest at home, focus on my recovery and do little but feed the baby, sleep and load up on nutritious food, herbals teas and smoothies (see Chapter 9, Nutrition). Perhaps not for the full 30 days, but certainly for as long as I feel like it.

Wendy Powell, a recognised maternal health expert and founder of MUTU System (which stands for mummy tummy), experienced life-threatening haemorrhages after the births of both her children. She felt bitter and let down by her body, but went on to use her experiences to better understand her clients:

'As wellness professionals, we are no different to the women we serve, and many of those who look like they've got it worked out feel it too: the rejection of our bodies for failing us during childbirth is all too common. Afterwards, we look down at the stretch marks and the overhang; we feel like our insides are going to fall out, and we shut down because it's just not feeling good anymore. I didn't appreciate the link between physical and mental health until I was in it. I remember sitting on the bathroom floor changing my baby's nappy, feeling utterly powerless and utterly exhausted, and bursting into tears. The shame that I felt, the indignation, the powerlessness, these feelings are all symptoms of a lack of education and truthful dialogue about what our bodies go through and what it feels like, coupled with the crazy expectations that we put on ourselves. Women who are fit and strong before birth are used to being able to control their bodies; getting out of the house to go for a run might be a form of self-care for them, and suddenly they can't do it. But instead of resting, healing and nurturing a body that's been

through an amazing feat and ordeal, too many women go into battle with it – "I will run despite the leaking, I will carry on regardless." I think that's a really sad place to be – and an awful lot of women are there.'

Sleep deprivation

Our sleep, health and behaviour are strongly linked. Matthew Walker, the author of *Why We Sleep*, is a British scientist who has spent his career researching sleep and what happens when we don't get enough. Through experiments at his sleep lab, he found that going for ten days on six hours of sleep a night – an amount most new mums consider a victory – leaves you as physically and mentally impaired as it does to go without sleep for 24 hours straight. Not getting enough sleep is as bad for your physical health as heavy drinking or regular smoking. And when we aren't getting enough sleep, we don't recognise it. Low-level exhaustion becomes an accepted norm, or baseline, he writes: 'Individuals fail to recognise how their perennial state of sleep deficiency has come to compromise their mental aptitude and physical vitality, including the slow accumulation of ill health.'

If you're not sleeping enough, you'll put on weight more easily, feel hungrier, and be more susceptible to illness. You'll also struggle to make memories or to learn anything new. In terms of your mental health, he says, sleep acts like therapy; if you're not getting eight hours you'll struggle to process emotional experiences, feel less creative, be quicker to show anger or rage, more susceptible to addiction and less able to balance out the ups and downs of a normal day. Given this, it's no surprise that so many of us end up in tears on the floor, weeping along with our infants, or feeling anger towards them. The next time you find yourself wailing along with your baby, wanting to throw something at your husband, or feeling like you can't do this anymore, try to take a deep breath and step back. The effects of even mild sleep deprivation are huge, and your body is dealing with so much more than just sleepless nights. For families with two or more babies, or a premature baby who needs to feed very frequently, the challenge of sleep can feel particularly acute.

> *Bridget found the illogical, circuitous thoughts that kept her awake at night started creeping into her days when sleep deprivation kicked in:*
> *'When you're not sleeping enough, the sort of thinking you do at night – when you can't stop your thoughts from escalating and going round in circles – creeps into your days, and it becomes harder to work out when you're being logical and when you're just being illogical and anxious. Next time, I'll be much more aware of this and ask myself, whenever I start worrying, is this day thinking or night thinking?'*

Getting more sleep

There is a whole industry built around this and I'm not going to compete with it. It's worth noting, however, that a lot of first-time mums say with hindsight that they became more controlling than usual after having a baby. As a result, they didn't always let their partners take decisions relating to the baby or let them do much to help, beyond changing nappies and preparing bottles. Women approaching their second children often say they'll be less controlling the next time around and will encourage their partners to do more. During the nights, we tend to take over, and it's not until we feel completely broken that we ask our partners to step in. If that sounds familiar, start sharing more of the work at night. If you've had a baby on your own, you probably won't have the option of sharing the tasks, particularly at night, and this can feel very hard and lonely – but nor will you have to worry about waking someone else up during the night, or sparking arguments because you or your partner is grumpy and fragile due to a lack of sleep.

It's hard to share the nights if you're exclusively breast-feeding, but you could express milk for one of the night feeds, or feed the baby first thing, then get your partner to get up with it while you go back to bed. If that doesn't work, you can still split the jobs so you go to bed early, while your partner stays up to finish any chores. And you can try to give yourself a regular nap time during the day. If you're bottle feeding, it's easier. Try to give each other a night off every now and again if you can, so that one of you sleeps in another room (again, with earplugs in or white noise, if necessary). And when the baby won't go down, make sure it's not always you who's soothing it. If you can share the burden in these early days and weeks, it will allow you to feel closer and help your partner to understand you better, prevent resentment building up in you (an emotion that can appear suddenly, without warning), allow them to build their own relation-ship with the baby, and make them feel better by being able to help. Partners often feel a lack of agency or a sense of dis-empowerment, out of their depth and unable to help. As one woman advised me, 'You shouldn't set up patterns with your baby that you don't want to keep. I set myself up as the primary care giver and the preferred parent, when that's not what either of us wanted.' If you can balance it a bit at the beginning, it may help you both in the long run.

A lot of mums regret acting like superheroes – trying to do the nights as well as the days and be the perfect mother who's keeping everyone and everything afloat. Becoming a parent can feel like being thrown into an unknowable universe, but if you can let go of the urge to know it all and be brilliant, accept that you're winging it and are just going to get by, you might find things fall into place more easily.

Sleep problems

I've heard women liken their postnatal sleep troubles to PTSD – they dream about sleep disturbances and wake to imaginary screams in the night. Start by doing what you can to keep anxiety out of the bedroom. Leaving your baby to cry for a few minutes isn't going to hurt them – in fact, it might even help teach them to soothe themselves. And, when you have a ghastly night, try not to catastrophise; yes, you'll be tired the next day, but you'll get through it.

Sweats – Oh, the night sweats. You wake up drenched in milk and hormones and fluids that your body is discharging through your pores. It can last for weeks, and some women say it's most noticeable around two weeks postpartum, as your oestrogen levels drop and your body rids itself of all unnecessary substances.

Sleep position – As a back-sleeper, I was desperate to return to sleeping face-up after the baby was born, but for the first few days it felt too strange; my uterus was still heavy, even though there was no baby in there. If you sleep on your front, you might struggle when your milk comes in and breasts start to feel engorged. For this reason, sleeping on your side as you did when pregnant may remain the most comfortable option. (Interestingly, co-sleeping used to be frowned upon but many health workers now recommend you feed your baby whilst lying down – with a bedside cot on their other side to prevent them falling out – so that if you do fall asleep from exhaustion, it doesn't matter – the baby will be safe, and you'll get more sleep.)

Insomnia – It's typical, the one night your baby sleeps like an angel, you lie awake worrying about something or waiting for the baby to wake up. Insomnia affects a lot of new mothers, even though they're in dire need of sleep. If it becomes anything more than occasional, however (clinically, insomnia is defined as occurring more than three nights a week), then it could be a symptom of postnatal mental-health issues. It's hard to decouple a problem from the normal anxieties that sometimes keep you awake at night, but if it persists and you're worried about the state of your mind, turn to a professional for help.

Thinking you don't need sleep – Believe it or not, feeling elated, as if you're nailing it as the ultimate supermum on very little sleep, is not necessarily a good sign either. If it feels like you're thriving on almost no sleep, it's possible that you have a mood disorder that is referred to medically as postnatal euphoria or hypomania, and that researchers say affects at least one in ten of us. If this sounds like you, read more in Chapter 10, and remember – everyone needs sleep.

9

Nutrition

If you are breastfeeding, the food you eat matters as much as it did when you were pregnant; you're still growing a baby, it's just on the outside, and your body also has a lot of healing to do. It's common to feel ravenous after giving birth; you've done something physically gruelling, you're suddenly producing milk, and your body needs all it can get to set about healing your tissues and restoring your balance. When I was pregnant, my husband used to nobly offer up his wine glass with the joke that he was drinking for two, but after I gave birth the joke was on him as he tried (and failed) to keep up with my meal requirements without putting on weight. This is the most nutritionally demanding time in a woman's life; you needed an extra 200 calories a day in the third trimester, but that shoots up to around 500 calories a day when you start breastfeeding. Stock your kitchen with nutritious snacks like fruit, nuts and seeds, and base your diet on whole, real foods like vegetables (leafy greens in particular), lentils and beans, full-fat dairy products, eggs, vegetables, and meat or vegan proteins like tofu, so that your body gets the nutrients it needs to heal and recalibrate.

Eating well can be expensive and time-consuming so the NHS recommends you look at frozen ingredients (often cheaper and quicker to prepare) and dried pulses (some of which don't need soaking and will cook quickly). If you eat meat, buy whole chickens rather than portions like legs and look for cheaper cuts like pork ribs or belly, beef brisket for slow cooking, and lamb scrag, which is great in a stew. Tinned fish like sardines are also packed with nutrients, and cheap.

'Warming' foods

From Jordan to China, Malaysia to the Amazon basin, traditional cultures around the world believe that postnatal women should consume only 'warm' food and drink for the first 30 to 40 days after the birth. Warm drinks is a self-explanatory concept – as a Brit, I don't need to be told of the advantages of tea over water – but what exactly does 'warm' food mean? It's not exactly vegan-friendly. Think soothing and nourishing; chicken or bone-broth soup, spices like cinnamon, turmeric and ginger, organ meats and eggs. Animal products tend to form the mainstay of traditional postpartum nutrition, while raw fruit and vegetables tend to be discouraged. In southwest China, this can extend to up to ten eggs per day, while in northern Brazil, it can mean nothing but boiled chicken for the first week.

Is there any evidence for why this practice of eating 'warm' foods, with an emphasis on animal products, exists the world over? I asked Lily Nichols, a renowned American dietician who specialises in pre- and postnatal nutrition. No, she says. First, she criticises the scientific cohort for not caring enough about postnatal women to do the research. Secondly, she says, this is a very tricky group of people to study. No one would put babies or mothers at risk if there were any potential downsides, and early motherhood is all-consuming. Even if researchers did manage to recruit study participants, how likely would they be to do what was asked of them? There is, however, a remarkable synchronicity between these traditional postpartum diets and what modern science dictates we should eat, she says – and one we shouldn't ignore. These 'warm' food diets are rich in proteins, iron, iodine, B vitamins, fats, zinc and choline, all of which are essential to rebuild the depleted mother and boost the quality of her breast milk.

What to eat

For many women, in terms of diet, the first trimester of pregnancy establishes a paradox: you want to be eating more healthily than ever, but all you feel like is stodge. The postpartum period can feel similarly unfair; just when you want to reclaim your body, it demands triple portions of everything. Although your diet may not be high on your priority list after having a baby, it should be, as should drinking water – you need a lot more water if you're breastfeeding, but studies also show that good hydration is important for healing tissue.

Protein – Protein is essential for repairing tissue damage, and it also helps to balance out blood sugar levels and prevent sugar cravings, which can help you to lose weight safely and sustainably. Adding protein (and good fats) to carb-based snacks is usually easy: if you're craving toast, have some avocado, a scrambled egg or nut butter on it. If it's muesli, put some full-fat natural yoghurt on it. Snack on cheese, nuts or seeds rather than biscuits. If you're vegan or vegetarian, the NHS says you need to pay special attention to your protein intake: you need plenty, from a variety of sources.

Iron – A recent review of research showed that around half of European women of childbearing age have 'small or depleted' iron stores, and pregnancy, birth and breastfeeding take a lot out of you, so it's safe to say that iron deficiency amongst new mums is common, and can cause fatigue, amongst other things. Your body can compensate for low iron levels by increasing the amount it absorbs, but dieticians recommend you eat plenty of iron-rich foods to help it.

Iron exists in animal products and vegetables, but iron from animal products – known as heme iron – is far more easily absorbed, and more effective due to the suite of other nutrients that come with it. Non-heme iron, which you'll get from dark leafy greens, grains and fortified foods, is complicated by the fact that a number of things can block its absorption, including the compounds found in tea, coffee and wine, and the calcium and proteins in milk products.

For an iron-rich treat, you could have a liver and bacon or lentil and soya-bean salad with peas, a heap of moules marinière (which are available pre-prepared in supermarkets), or a snack of pumpkin seeds. As a safety net, nutritionists recommend you take an iron supplement, particularly if you're not regularly eating organ meats or shellfish (which some people don't like and could work out to be rather expensive). Ferrous bisglycinate is popular because it has minimal side-effects.

Easy to digest – Look for foods that are gentle on your digestive system. Your organs are still moving around and your digestive system might not be in the best shape. This may be why, in the Far East, women eat soup after giving birth – it is both nourishing and gentle.

Fibre – Eat high-fibre foods, especially if you've had any trouble with constipation or haemorrhoids: ground linseed (flaxseed), oats, wholegrain carbs and, as a general rule, fruits beginning with the letter 'p' – peaches, plums, pears, pineapple, papaya and, of course, prunes – or their juice.

Vitamin D – If you're breastfeeding, you're advised to take a vitamin D supplement of 10 micrograms each day, because your baby is using your reserves to build up its own. A general postnatal vitamin should include this as well as the other key nutrients you might be missing.

Vitamin B12 – Vitamin B12 is essential for you and your baby; it's found in animal products like fish, meat, poultry, eggs and dairy, but doesn't exist in plant foods, so if you're following a strict vegetarian or vegan diet, you should consider taking a supplement. (See Chapter 19 for guidance on how much you need.)

Vitamin C and antioxidants – Your immune system may not be as strong as usual as you're still in recovery and not getting the sleep your body needs. For vitamin C, eat plenty of dark green leafy vegetables, kiwis, grapefruit and oranges. Kiwis are vitamin C powerhouses – just one contains around three-quarters of your recommended daily intake. For antioxidants like beta carotene that also support the immune system, eat orange squashes like pumpkins and root vegetables such as sweet potato.

Fats – Even if you're keen to start losing weight, don't avoid fats: healthy fats from nuts, seeds, avocados, coconut and coconut milk, olive oil, cheese and oily fish will balance out sugar cravings and provide essential nutrients for your recovery.

> *Acupuncturist Ross J. Barr believes iron deficiency is a widespread – and often undiagnosed – problem, and has seen clients recover with just a simple iron supplement: 'I'm always surprised by how blood loss and subsequent anaemia caused by childbirth aren't given more focus. The parameters for blood deficiency in this country are kind of World War II era; if you're not fainting or don't have some sort of blood clotting going on, no one cares too much. In other countries, the parameters for what constitutes iron deficiency are much narrower. It's crazy how many women I see who have been prescribed drugs for depression or anxiety when actually they're anaemic; the symptoms are very similar. Rather than anti-depressants, they just need a good iron supplement like Floradix or an improved diet.'*

When will I lose the weight?

You shouldn't try to lose weight in the early weeks and months – your uterus is shrinking, your breasts are settling down and your blood volume is declining. If you're breast-feeding, enjoy the fact that it burns around 500 calories per day and that Brazilian supermodel Gisele Bünchen swears by it. If you develop a voracious appetite, don't fight it – it's nature's way of giving you what you need.

Rather than think about losing weight now, nutrition-ists and personal trainers suggest you consider a nine-month timeline – nine months on, nine months off. This, they say, is a sensible timeframe within which most people can lose their excess weight, although for some it takes much longer and the extra weight can linger until you stop breastfeeding (see Chapter 19).

Caffeine

After nine months of prohibition, I quickly lost all self-control when it came to my old daytime drug of choice. One month in, a typical morning involved a dirty nappy, a cup of tea whilst breastfeeding, another dirty nappy, another cup of tea, breakfast, another cup of tea, tidying up while the baby napped, another breakfast (with tea), waking the baby and having one last cup (decaf this time) before leaving the house. Tea became my main source of hydration and raison d'être, supplemented by good food, which was one of the few things to transition with us from our old, childless life into this unknown realm; Philip cooked lavish suppers because he felt he didn't have much else to do. He fed me, I fed the baby.

Technically, I should not have been consuming litres of Yorkshire tea whilst breastfeeding. Caffeine does cross into breastmilk and can mess up your baby's sleep – but research suggests you need to drink quite a lot for it to do so. The UK guidelines propose a maximum of 300 milligrams of caffeine per day. That's at least six cups of tea (or one or two Americano coffees), I would tell myself, as I put the kettle on again.

The other problem with caffeine is that it affects your own ability to sleep. The typical advice is to sleep when your baby sleeps – but it's hard to nap at 11 a.m. with three cups of builders' brew inside you. Roughly 12 hours after you have a caffeinated drink, a quarter of that caffeine is still circulating in your body. As Matthew Walker explains in his book, *Why We Sleep*, caffeine masks tiredness by blocking and inactivating the receptors in your brain that would otherwise receive messages instructing your body to go to sleep. It is, he says, akin to 'sticking your fingers in your ears to shut out a sound'. It can mess with your ability to nap and get to sleep at night, and reduce the amount of deep sleep you get during the night. Walker recommends cutting off caffeine around 12 to 14 hours before you want to go to sleep. This explains why I struggled to nap and why, if you're aiming to catch up on some sleep in the daytime, you may need to say that caffeine is off-limits.

10

Mental Health

Motherhood has a dark side. For some of us, that manifests in fleeting moments of despair; for others, the darkness is far more serious and entrenched. It's an uncomfortable fact but suicide is the leading cause of death in new mums, which is why GPs and midwives have focused on improving postnatal mental health in recent years.

The author Clover Stroud likens motherhood to being pixelated, 'because it feels like you're being shattered into pieces.' If you can't find ways to hold those pieces together, to give some shape to your life, it can become hard to keep going. With the right support, however, mothers come through it and finish their journey more resilient and with greater self-awareness than ever before.

A number of the women I interviewed likened post-natal depression to grief; as if they needed to grieve for the life they'd had. I didn't have postnatal depression, but I can still identify with this. After the initial high of birth and meeting my baby, I went through a long and gradual process of coming to terms with it. As you make this transition, you have to deal with all sorts of new emotions and challenges: the ambivalence of needing to be close to your child but craving physical and mental space; the ideals of motherhood that we try to live up to but that leave us feeling guilty or like we've failed; and the effect that this tiny new being has on our existing relationships, which is huge and impossible to quantify.

Dr Genevieve von Lob, a mother, clinical psychologist and author of *Happy Parent, Happy Child*, explains that when you're tired and can't think straight, you revert to unhelpful old patterns and scripts – which might include being harsher than usual on yourself, listening to negative voices running away with things in your head, comparing yourself to others, or simply not feeling good enough. 'It just gets magnified as a parent, particularly when you're a new mum,' she said. Von Lob's advice is to do anything that takes you out of your head, even if it's just for a minute: stretch, listen to music, meditate or, when you're ready, walk or swim. 'Learn to observe your thoughts rather than get caught up in them, and try to speak to yourself as gently and kindly as possible.'

Nicky, a successful accountant who had postnatal depression after a difficult birth, wants more women to be open about the pressures and psychological shifts that becoming a mother demands:
'Women feel so much societal and cultural pressure to love motherhood and to feel like they love their children instantly. There's a spectrum of emotions – we all have ambivalence – and it's important for people to know that's OK. I didn't have any visceral, hormonal feelings towards my baby for months. You don't know this little thing, after all, you don't understand what they want, and you're so massively tired and exhausted sometimes you just haven't got anything to give. So many women put pressure on themselves to be these perfect mothers and to feel positive about parenting all of the time, and it just isn't real.'

Baby blues

The baby blues, as it's commonly known, affects up to 80 per cent of us and kicks in a few days after the birth. During pregnancy, a lot of us feel great because our hormones are running high, stimulating endorphins that act like morphine, dulling our perceptions of pain and upping our positivity. By day three postpartum, however, your hormone levels are as low as they will ever be, other than during the menopause. When you add sleep deprivation to this, it may explain why you suddenly feel like you're married to an ogre, your baby is somehow not right, or you just want to curl up in bed and cry. A lack of sleep raises levels of cortisol, the stress hormone, so will make you more easily stressed. If these feelings don't go away within a week or two, talk to your healthcare team. The baby blues didn't hit me, and I suspect this is because we all slept pretty well on our first few nights as a family; for us, the sleep deprivation kicked in a little later.

To ease the symptoms, sleep as much as you possibly can. Try to ensure that your partner, a friend or family member is helping out with your share of the chores, and ask someone else to look after the baby so you can spend some time alone. Tell your partner what's going on with your body; explain that you're falling down a physiological rock face as your hormone levels nosedive. Tell them you're on the ultimate post-festival come-down, if that will help them to understand. And talk to friends and family who are mums and can help; a lot of women go on a journey of discovery in these first few weeks, and they are often happy – sometimes eager – to talk about it.

Olivia Inge, a holistic medical practitioner and former catwalk model, recalls giving herself points if she managed to achieve certain tasks in a day:

'In terms of depression, there are a few key things to look for to gauge how you are coping. One of them is how you deal with personal hygiene and whether you let it fall by the wayside. I used to give myself points if I managed to brush my teeth, have a shower, change my t-shirt; little things that might seem inconsequential but really matter. If you let something slip, you need to ask why. Another thing to look out for is being afraid to leave your baby with someone else, or finding your sleep starts to suffer because you're always checking on the baby. And then there's the lack of desire to do common tasks, like eat, sleep, be around people or leave the house. Being aware of these behaviours can be a useful predictor of your mental state. If you feel wobbly, let someone know, so they can help you to feel more secure in your mind and therefore in your role as a mum.'

Baby brain

I never liked the term 'baby brain' – I found it condescending. I objected to the idea that, because I was pregnant or had a baby, I should be somehow mentally deficient. I worked like mad during my pregnancy, publishing a story that I'd been researching for months just ten days before my due date. I even did some editing work – from the sofa, I should add – in the first few weeks of my son's life. It wasn't particularly good work, but I did it.

I later discovered, however, that I was wrong: baby brain is a defined thing and not, as I had assumed, a cute term for women who are so sleep-deprived, fed up or out of their mind with boredom that their brain ceases to function. For two years after you have your baby, your brain will be smaller in parts, having undergone a pruning process during pregnancy that primes it for maximum empathy and bonding (as covered in more detail in Part 1). When I attempted to use an unusual word in the weeks after my baby was born, I often found that the word would simply evade me. Gaping, open-mouthed, I would reach for it helplessly, and then eventually feel obliged to fill the silence with something else. But the result was not always coherent. Because of this, I learned not to be ambitious in conversation.

Interestingly, some doctors and scientists believe the hormonal changes that take place during this period actually increase your IQ, making you more intelligent than before. I'm dubious of how well I'd have fared on an IQ test in the weeks after the baby was born, but I do wonder whether these brain changes could have explained my new superpower: being able to wake from an apparently deep sleep in the middle of the night whenever my baby smacked his lips in polite, near-silent warning that he would like a little milk soon. The technical term for this is hypervigilance, when your senses are heightened to look after your offspring. In milliseconds, I would shake off slumber and be up, breasts surging and ready to feed. These structural brain changes may also explain why we as new mothers cry such a lot.

Crying

Crying deserves a special mention because it's such a universal characteristic of early motherhood, and not something everyone is used to. At first, you cry with elation. Next, you cry with exhaustion. And then you cry with desperation and defeat – because months have gone by and there's no end in sight.

Crying is a normal and healthy response to the unique pressures that accompany having a newborn baby, and can help to release stress and gain a sense of relief, says Dr Genevieve von Lob. But you can also reach such a state of exhaustion that you find yourself crying a lot more than usual, without feeling any better – a sign that you may be in need of more support. The trick, von Lob says, is to get to know yourself well enough to distinguish between normal, healthy crying, and tears that show you are suffering from anxiety or depression.

Dr Genevieve von Lob, clinical psychologist, on the importance of crying:
'A lot of us have been conditioned to hold back our tears, but crying puts us in touch with our emotions. For much of my life, I struggled to connect with my tears, and I would suppress the urge to cry. But I knew that allowing myself to let go was the only way to experience how I was really feeling deep down inside. I can understand why so many women find the prospect of allowing the tears to flow so overwhelming, since so many of us have felt that we have to wear a mask and keep our most powerful feelings hidden. Sometimes, women are reluctant to cry because – rightly or wrongly – they fear the men around them will feel helpless and won't know what to do or say. We can all help new mothers by giving them space to experience whatever emotions are coming up without fear of being judged or having to manage other people's feelings.'

Anxiety

Postnatal anxiety is just as common as postnatal depression; it affects roughly one in ten and ranges from mild to severe. You might find that worries and fears dominate your thinking, you feel constantly on edge, struggle with getting to sleep, feel responsible for problems, or experience physical effects like panic attacks or a racing heartbeat. The fear that you're losing your mind can be made worse by lack of sleep, unruly hormones and the physical and mental demands on you and your time.

Breastfeeding is a common cause of anxiety, particularly during the early weeks when your milk is establishing and you are working things out. In 2019, a team of American researchers found that postnatal anxiety was linked to a lower uptake and shorter duration of breastfeeding. Women with anxiety were also more likely to supplement with formula or just stop breastfeeding altogether. It's unclear whether the anxiety causes women to stop breastfeeding, or whether it's problematic breastfeeding that causes the anxiety in the first place, but there is a link between the two (see also Imogen's story about psychological transitions on page 325).

While science hasn't yet established whether anxiety means you make less milk, many women believe it does. If you feel that breastfeeding isn't going well, however, then not being anxious is easier said than done. Again, talk to other mums – you'll be surprised how many have their own story about breastfeeding and would like to have stern words with Leonardo da Vinci and his ilk for painting such idyllic pictures of babies at their mothers' breasts.

If your anxiety is mild, work out what you need to ground yourself – whether it's yoga, time to cook, a walk, time alone, or talking to friends – and make it an absolute priority, on a regular basis, to keep yourself well. If your anxiety feels insurmountable, make an appointment to see your doctor, who can prescribe talking therapy, self-help programmes and medication (see Chapter 23 for more on anxiety and mental health). And if you don't want to see a doctor, try at least to open up a conversation about it with someone you trust.

Postnatal depression

In over 80 per cent of cases, postnatal depression starts within the first six weeks of childbirth, so now is the time to look out for yourself and to ask those around you to do the same, particularly if you have had mental health issues in the past; a 2014 study by the British Medical Council found that over 80 per cent of women with postnatal depression already had a history of depression. The chemical changes in your brain after birth are known to trigger mood swings and symptoms of postnatal depression. On top of this, you might not be getting enough rest in order to recover from the birth. Sleep deprivation (see Chapter 8, Rest and Sleep) can further exacerbate the symptoms and, in somewhere between one in seven and one in ten women, these symptoms develop into actual postnatal depression.

Other risk factors include having a difficult birth or caesarean, difficulty breastfeeding, if there are any physical problems with your baby, or if you are isolated or stressed. A recent study suggests that women who had severe morning sickness, known as hyperemesis gravidarum, are also at a higher risk of developing postnatal depression: a 2020 study found that nearly 30 per cent of women with hyperemesis went on to have postnatal depression, compared with just 6 per cent of women without the condition, making them four times more likely to suffer from it.

Farah, a GP and mother of two, suffered mild postnatal depression after an emergency caesarean, with a baby that wouldn't stop crying:

'I think I was a bit depressed after I had my first, which wasn't surprising because I had an emergency caesarean section at 35 weeks; risks for post-natal depression include premature delivery, unplanned emergency caesarean section and having a difficult birth, amongst other things. I don't think I acknowledged that I was depressed, and I don't think I was very depressed, but I did struggle. I got a congratulations letter from a cousin who'd had a baby a few months before and sent me a photo of her baby. She obviously was loving being a mother: "Oh it's so wonderful, and, how great you can spend all this lovely time, here's a picture of my darling snuggle-pumpkin." And I was looking at the photo of this happy baby, and I was looking at mine – a screaming, angry, never-sleeping, constantly-feeding baby – and I thought, no, that's not a lovely snuggle-pumpkin, it's a horrible, cross, boiled goblin. How do you enjoy a baby? I'm not enjoying babies, I thought.'

The Edinburgh Postnatal Depression Scale is the standard yardstick that doctors use to screen for postnatal depression. It is widely available online if you (or a friend or partner) think you have reason to worry. Symptoms include losing interest in your world and no longer enjoying things that once gave you pleasure, feeling tired but having trouble sleeping, struggling to concentrate or make decisions, having an increased or decreased appetite, feelings of helplessness and guilt, and blaming yourself for things that have happened. You may also worry about not feeling a bond to your baby, or imagine hurting him or her – thoughts that can be terrifying, but that rarely come to anything. Some women also think about harming themselves or even committing suicide. On top of all of this, your partner may experience depression as well (see Part 4).

A question that is useful to ascertain whether you might be suffering from depression is, are you enjoying your baby? You can also ask whether your negative emotions are affecting your ability to care for yourself or your baby. If they are, talking therapy can help, as well as medication that is safe to use while breastfeeding and can correct the chemical imbalance. Even though doctors still fail to diagnose thousands of cases of postnatal depression every year, the pathways for treating it have improved vastly, so you should be fast-tracked to someone who can help.

At the start of her pregnancy, Nicky was on a low dose of anti-depressants for mild anxiety and depression but came off them and felt fine, until a traumatic birth involving a failed attempt to turn her breech baby at around 40 weeks culminated in an emergency caesarean, and she developed severe postnatal depression:
'Everything seemed like it was going wrong. The birth didn't go to plan. Then breastfeeding wasn't working; I drove myself into the ground trying to get him to breastfeed. I got to ten days postnatal and reached breaking point; I was absolutely done. I sobbed to my husband "I hate being a mum." I said, "these are the worst ten days of my life. Why won't he breastfeed, why can't it just be natural? I don't want to sleep in the same room as him tonight, I don't want to do this."
'The next day I went to see a doctor for an emergency appointment. He said you've had a series of traumatic events, let's not rush to label this as postnatal depression and to

medicate this, telling me I needed family support and rest. It was a poor decision, to send away a new mum who's saying, I don't want to be here, without offering medication and psychological support. After that, I became obsessive and had a fascination with my baby's bout of eczema; I obsessed about his skin and felt that I'd done something to cause it. I didn't want anyone to see my baby because of his eczema – his skin wasn't "normal" in my mind and I was catastrophising that it would never get better. I was suicidal by this point. I kept saying I just don't want this life, over and over again. I was trapped, with no attachment or bond; it felt like the worst mistake of my life. I didn't think I had postnatal depression but that motherhood was just like this. I thought the baby was the cause of my depression, it was never going to get better, and the only possible solution was to remove myself from the situation. Mentally, I didn't know you could be in so much pain.

'A month later, I was back at the doctors' surgery. The doctors had no idea how to handle postnatal depression of this severity. They told me to go on a very low dose of antidepressant medication but didn't offer any other support. If you have somebody who's suicidal, sleep-deprived and has a young child, putting them on such a low dose of medication, without offering other support like a referral to a psychiatrist or a therapist, is dangerous; I very nearly ended my life on it. I ended up going to A&E because my doctor didn't know what to do. I spoke to a lovely mental health nurse, they upped my meds, and I started seeing a crisis team of mental health support workers. But I needed specialist perinatal care and that didn't exist where I lived. Things became so bad that I nearly acted on a plan to end my life. After that, I went into a mother and baby unit. I was 30 years old, a *high-functioning, together person with a career and lots of family and friends and a healthy lifestyle, and I'd disintegrated to nothing. In hospital, I had this awful experience, known as "the void", when I went past sadness and being low to the point that there was nothing there. I went into a chasm of nothingness. Then, with support, medication and therapy, this really gradual process of recovery happened, like a grief cycle, and I eventually found ways to manage the pain. Postnatal depression is like grief – for the life you had, for the expectations you had, and for the motherhood and relationship with your baby that you'd imagined. We talk about adolescence and how the transition into adulthood can be really hard emotionally and psychologically for teenagers, but becoming a parent is such a huge psychological shift, such a mentally and physically demanding time, and it's just not talked about.'*

Birth trauma

Birth trauma is considered shorthand for symptoms of post-traumatic stress disorder as a result of childbirth, and it's sadly becoming more, not less, common in the UK. The cause can be the sort of event that would traumatise anyone – believing that your or your baby's life is in serious danger, for instance – but also less clear-cut things, like feeling out of control, losing your dignity, not being listened to, or being subject to medical procedures without your consent. It can affect the woman who wants a caesarean but is given an induction, the woman who a doctor compels to walk half-naked through a labour ward, and the woman a doctor leaves alone with her feet in stirrups and an open door. Academics at City University in London recently estimated that around one in 25 women end up with PTSD after birth, although many more likely experience some symptoms. The Birth Trauma Association believes that around 200,000 women (representing almost 30 per cent of all births) feel the impact of birth trauma in the UK each year.

You may find you start reliving aspects of what happened, through flashbacks, recurrent thoughts, nightmares, physical symptoms like pain and nausea, or finding any reminder of it intensely distressing. You might find you need to avoid anything that could potentially remind you of it, feel like you have to keep busy, blank out details of what happened, feel emotionally and physically detached from yourself and your body, or be unable to express affection. You might find you're hypervigilant, constantly alert, irritable and easily startled, or worry that something is going to happen to your baby. And you may just find you feel unhappy or low, blame yourself for the birth, or just blank it out.

Getting help

If your trauma symptoms are mild, the NHS recommends taking a 'watchful waiting' approach – wait and see, basically – for around four weeks, because two in every three people who have problems after a traumatic experience get better on their own.

Experiencing upsetting feelings is normal if you experienced a difficult birth. For a lot of people the first step is to find someone sympathetic and understanding to confide in. This could be anyone from your midwife to your partner or mum. Take care of yourself – eat well, sleep as much as you possibly can, then ask someone to help you get more sleep, establish routines, and make time to relax.

You can consider contacting your hospital and asking them to go through your medical records with you, which you are legally entitled to see. When it's done well, a debrief by a doctor or midwife on exactly what happened can be very helpful (see Jemima's story on page 140). However, it's not always done well, and NICE does not currently recommend it: 'The systematic provision to that individual alone of brief, single-session interventions (often referred to as debriefing) that focus on the traumatic incident should not be routine practice when delivering services,' its guidelines state.

If your symptoms do persist or worsen, you may need professional support, and the two treatments currently recommended by NICE are Trauma-focused Cognitive Behavioural Therapy (CBT) and EMDR (Eye Movement Desensitization and Reprocessing – see page 139). Accessing them on the NHS, however, is not always easy.

While some people are lucky and live in a part of the country where they have access to quality perinatal mental health care on the health service, for others it's tricky, says Alex Heath, a clinical hypnotherapist and midwife trainer specialising in birth trauma. Alex had her two babies at home, and when she started working as a doula and had her first experience of a labour ward, she was shocked; midwives themselves were often full of fear, and even those who joined the profession because they wanted to make birth better had become part of a system that, she felt, could be dehumanising and cruel in its treatment of women. She later discovered that mental health problems are common amongst midwives, many of whom suffer burnout, depression, anxiety and PTSD as a result of their experiences. Research conducted in Australia showed that as many as 33 per cent of midwives had Secondary Traumatic Stress as a result of what they'd witnessed.

Alex urges anyone struggling with symptoms, whether physical or mental, to get help – even if it means finding a way to pay for it, which may be a daunting prospect. 'We've been brought up with the NHS always being there for us when really bad things happen. We have an expectation that it'll be there for this – and that's just not always the case,' she says. If you are on a low income or are struggling financially, don't write off private care just yet – many therapists offer a reduced rate, and some will even ask you to pay whatever you can afford.

Alex offers the following advice:

Acknowledge – If you had a difficult birth or struggled in the weeks afterwards, it is very important to acknowledge what you've been through. Just because you have friends who've suffered the same thing, it doesn't mean it's right or acceptable. If you still feel upset by your birth, or the care you received, then that is not OK and you can do something about it. If somebody says, 'it's very normal – birth is difficult', or, 'at least you've got a healthy baby', or any other refrain that diminishes your experience, their comments are a reflection of their inadequacies and not yours. You need to really acknowledge what you've been through.

Be compassionate – Be kind to yourself. Imagine your best friend had just gone through what you have. How would you help her? Often, women blame themselves for a negative birth experience, especially if they feel regret about something. Being compassionate to yourself is very important.

Be persistent – The double onslaught of psychological and physical symptoms after birth can be so overwhelming that

Mental Health

it makes it very hard to ask for what you need in terms of health care, or to even know or identify what you need. If you suspect you could benefit from professional help – either physiotherapy, psychological support or both – ask for it and be tenacious. As Alex says, 'Often women are vulnerable to receiving poor or coercive care because they have been brought up to be good girls and do what they're told. They want to be cared for, and feel they have to acquiesce to get that care.' If you need something from your doctor, don't take no for an answer, she says. If things don't feel right, you don't have to tolerate it. Dig deep within yourself, or ask someone for help with getting help.

Trauma-focused Cognitive Behavioural Therapy (CBT)

Over a course of sessions, a therapist will help you come to terms with a traumatic event. This might involve asking you to confront it and then think about the memories in detail. The therapist helps you to manage your distress, but also helps you to correct unhelpful thoughts or feelings, for example, blaming yourself for something that is not your fault. In this way, they allow you to take control of your negative emotions by repositioning the experience in your mind.

EMDR

EMDR (Eye Movement Desensitization and Reprocessing) sounds a bit cuckoo. I'd heard about it because a friend had used it to get over the trauma of witnessing ethnic cleansing in Myanmar. The basic premise is quite simple. With close supervision from a trained therapist, you picture a scene that represents your traumatic event, then you let your brain explore it whilst doing a series of movements; usually either tapping the right then left side of your body, or following a moving hand left and right with your eyes. These left/right movements allow the rational, grown-up side of your brain, the left, to 'talk', metaphorically speaking, to the right, which contains the trauma. As you think about your experience and allow yourself to explore it in all its depth and complexity, new neural pathways form that enable you to process the memory so it's no longer traumatic.

Therapists need to be trained and accredited to offer EMDR. The treatment is safe and effective whether you do it weeks after the traumatic event takes place, or many years down the line. People often describe it as very emotionally draining and find the process itself upsetting. For this reason, you need to start with a baseline of feeling secure and supported. Therapists warn of two common misconceptions: firstly, that the treatment consists only of the memory processing stage, when you do the tapping or eye movements. The preparation that comes before this, including recognising past trauma as well as positive life experiences, is essential, even if it might feel irrelevant at times. Secondly, people mistakenly think that the experience of EMDR will be so distressing that it's not for them. The memory processing stage can be very upsetting, but you should feel safe and reassured throughout.

Jemima's waters broke and, 24 hours later, midwives began an induction, ignoring her protestations that she wanted a caesarean. Only when the induction failed, she was septic and her baby was in distress, did she get the caesarean, by which point she was hallucinating about her own death:

'*I do not remember the birth of my son. All in all, it was incredibly traumatic, followed by a missed infection, anaemia, jaundice and not getting the support I needed to breastfeed. By the time I left hospital after six days, my boobs were already ruined and in agony. I then had to deal with not being able to breastfeed, which sent me into a deep depression. I could never have imagined the emotional and physical pain that trying to breastfeed and failing every time would bring. I thought I would never bond with my boy. However, there is a happy ending to this.*

'*I booked in for a debrief at the hospital after friends who had had traumatic births told me I needed to push for this. When I went, I realised that all the things I started to think hadn't really happened, actually had. It was affirming, and it made me realise that the start my son and I had was not my fault; that I couldn't blame myself.*

'*We saw a midwife two weeks after the birth who picked up that I was not coping. She signposted me to postnatal counselling. At five weeks, I was diagnosed with birth-related PTSD. I had many weeks of counselling; I was so thankful for that service. The GP was also acutely aware of what we had been through and kept an eye on us. Talking is such a key part of the recovery process, even though it's incredibly painful. It made me see that I cared incredibly deeply for my son, even though I felt like I was a terrible mother and he deserved better.*

'*I put a formal complaint in to the hospital. Those who know me know I am not a complainer! However, I knew that I didn't want any other women, babies and families to go through what I did. So many women don't know where to start with this; but just put pen to paper. I have now met with the hospital, who have been very open and honest with me about the failings in my case and changes they are making to their services. A traumatic birth can't be changed but you can drive change so it stops happening to others.*

'As for me and my little boy, where to even begin? I cried every single day until he was four and a half months old. I lived in a constant state of anxiety, thinking, "I just need to keep him alive and well, as I've failed him to this point." I saw all these other mothers who seemed to be having a great time, talking about the rushes of love. I spent so many hours, days, weeks and months in deep heartbreak about not breastfeeding and having no bond. But I could not have been more wrong. I wish I could have seen how it would be in the future, so I could have been more kind to myself. Now, ten months in, we are so close – but at the time I could never have imagined it feeling this way.'

Postnatal hypomania or euphoria

Postnatal euphoria or hypomania is a mood disorder where a new mother feels on top of the world, like superwoman, with no need to sleep or rest – which would be ideal if it didn't often lead to a period of irritability, anxiety or depression afterwards, which occasionally turns into a mild form of bipolar disorder. Perinatal mental health experts at the University of Birmingham believe that this common condition affects at least one in ten women after childbirth – but it is virtually unheard of. 'It should not be assumed that women who are feeling elated, coping on little sleep and/or feeling like "super-mum" are at low risk of requiring postpartum support,' Professor Femi Oyebode, head of psychiatry at the university, and his colleague Jessica Heron wrote in their 2011 review of the subject. On the contrary, postnatal hypomania – facetiously dubbed the 'baby pinks' – could be a flag for future depression or anxiety. The symptoms – racing thoughts, talking quickly, being very active, struggling to concentrate, acting impulsively, not needing much sleep and being irritable – are hard to separate from the normal happiness of a new baby and don't usually require treatment, unless you have a history of bipolar disorder or psychosis or develop more severe mania, anxiety or depression with time.

Maria, whose father is bipolar, experienced 'hyper-happiness' after the birth of her daughter, which turned out to be a precursor to postnatal anxiety:
'In the first three months, I had the opposite of depression – baby euphoria. It all felt so unknowable and beautiful and incredible at first, but I didn't feel like I knew what I was doing. Anything we did was like, that's amazing, we just did that! I didn't feel that sleepy contentment, I felt like a superhero. How did I get through that? I'd ask myself; I'm so incredible. But, really, what was I doing other than feeding my baby on the sofa and watching TV? It was a hyper-happiness. And I wasn't putting a premium on sleep. People say to sleep when the baby sleeps, but I was like, fuck you – I'm going for a run. And despite very little sleep, I felt amazingly happy and overwhelmed with joy. But it was an escalating cycle, and sleep deprivation was a massive factor in my becoming completely untethered. We think that my dad developing bipolar disorder was precipitated by sleep deprivation; I've actually felt like I was replaying patterns of his at times. Were I to do it again, I'd be very careful to get four-hour stretches of sleep every night, prioritising sleep rather than embracing the highs and lows that little sleep brings.'

Postpartum psychosis

This is an acute mental illness characterised by hallucinations, delusions and severe depression that affects around one in every 1,000 new mums (0.1 per cent) and is considered a medical emergency, so you need to get help immediately. It can be frightening for everyone involved and the most severe symptoms can last for weeks or more, but women usually recover fully with no lasting damage to their relationship with their baby – although it can take time to rebuild confidence in yourself and come to terms with what has happened.

Postpartum psychosis usually starts suddenly within two weeks of you having your baby, and often in the first few days. It is rare, but possible, for it to start several weeks after the baby is born. Symptoms are different for everyone but they include mania (a high, euphoric mood), depression, confusion, hallucinations and delusions, and they can change rapidly. The Royal College of Psychiatrists' website gives a comprehensive list of symptoms.

Doctors don't know exactly why it happens, but they believe it's a combination of factors including genes and family history; you are more likely to get postpartum psychosis if a close relative has had it. Hormone levels and sleep disturbances may also play a part. And some people are just more predisposed to it than others, in particular people with bipolar disorder type I and schizoaffective disorder. If you are high risk, it's important that you tell everyone who's involved in your care, so they can plan for the support you may need.

If symptoms emerge and you already have a mental health care team, or have a contact number for your local mental health or crisis service, call them immediately. If not, see your GP or midwife on the same day, call 111, or go to A&E. If they send you away but your symptoms get worse, go back to be reassessed because the situation can change very quickly. Ideally, women with postpartum psychosis are treated in specialist mother and baby units, where they receive the psychiatric care they need while staff help them care for their babies. These are, however, limited, so you may go to a general psychiatric ward until a bed becomes available or until you are well enough to care for your baby.

Hannah, a professional woman in her early thirties, had never had any mental health issues until her induction at 42 weeks ended in a traumatic forceps delivery:
'The timeline between her being born and breathing is really vivid – it took 90 seconds – and I remember wondering, is she going to live? She was taken off to intensive care and it was just David and me left in the room. I knew something had happened to me, but there was no baby and nobody around. When my mum got to me, I was still covered in blood, so she washed me – like reverting to childhood. We were in hospital for about five days; the baby was upstairs, I was downstairs, and they would call me up to breastfeed her. The focus was all on the baby; no one asked me, are you alright about everything? All the while the nurses were saying, she's not really bonding with that baby. I stopped sleeping because every time I closed my eyes this loop of nightmares started. By the time we got home, I already couldn't think straight, and on about day 12 David started asking people for advice. He was met with a unison of voices saying, it's fine, this is what happens to women when they have babies, they just go a bit loopy. He had a real problem getting anybody to engage.
'In the end, he got a midwife sent round. By this point, I was not sleeping at all, and thought I was in labour again. The midwife said to him, I think your wife has something

called postpartum psychosis and we need to get her to the doctor. David told me we were going to the doctor for himself. I totally understand why he did that, but I was quite delusional and it added to my confusion. The doctor gave David a letter, and he and my dad took me to A&E. It felt like I was being held captive and I didn't understand why. Many hours later, we saw a psychiatrist. By then I was very scared and defensive; my flight mode had ignited and heightened my hysteria. I got upset and stressed, and they started trying to offer me drugs, but I wasn't interested. It all culminated in me getting sectioned.

'I was transferred to a psychiatric ward in King's College, where I'd given birth, but this time without the baby. Whether something was real or not real was a big thing in my head as I tried to piece together what was going on. David had promised he wouldn't leave me, but then they asked him to step out of the room and told him he had to go; being torn apart was just awful. It was everything you'd imagine of a mental ward; so surreal. I was there for two days and nights, stuck in this loop of trying to remember my name and figure out who I was. Meanwhile, my family were banging on doors trying to get me out. Eventually, I was taken to a specialist mother and baby unit, where I had the baby with me. I had this obsession that all the people around me were actors. I was telling everyone I was fine, and that David had put me in this mental institute. This made it a big challenge for him because people were saying, I don't think it's as big as you're making out.

'Breastfeeding went off the table as soon as they started medicating me. I was given an antipsychotic, which basically zombified me; I'd say I lost a year of my life to it. I was discharged after almost two months but relapsed a few weeks later. At that point, I felt completely and utterly saddened by

everything and didn't have any energy to push on. It wasn't until they told me they were going to prescribe electroconvulsive therapy that I woke up; I really didn't want it. I don't know whether I dug deep, but somehow I got better without it. I went back to work when my daughter turned one, but then had another relapse. I hadn't dealt with anything that had happened – the trauma of the birth – so there was a lot to talk about. I ended up hospitalised again, but it gave me the time to talk through everything. I don't know when is the right time to talk about your birth and what happens to your body and your mind, but having gone through that process again when I was ready was really beneficial. Realistically, it wasn't until she had her third birthday that there was enough water under the bridge to say I'm over it, this is the real deal now.'

11

Wee and Poo

'Nervous.' 'Terrified.' 'Like I was going to burst my stitches.' 'As if my insides were going to fall out.' 'I will never, ever, ever do a poo again.' This is how women have described to me their misgivings about their first poo after having a baby – and these feelings of trepidation are not helpful. By building up a simple poo into an agonising rite of passage, a key scene in the tragicomedy of early motherhood, women can make it worse for themselves. Pain is not really pain per se, but the brain's interpretation of it, and if the brain expects something to be incredibly painful, it's more likely that it will be. If you allow the tension to build up, your first poo probably will be painful. And if you ignore the 'call to stool', as one physio puts it, your brain may just stop hearing the messages and you'll end up with a new problem – constipation. You need to coax your brain and bowel into realising that a movement won't be painful. Relax. 'Defecate without fear!' as one delightful interviewee put it. Such is the power of the brain over the body that, if you can do that, it really won't be so bad. If you have stitches and opening your bowels puts pressure on them, you can hold a clean pad against the perineum and press gently as you poo to support them. Your stitches should hold up, and the worst will probably be that you have to wait a while, or pop a haemorrhoid or two back in when you're done. If you've had a serious tear – a bad second-, or a third- or fourth-degree tear – you'll likely be advised to take laxatives to make it easier to go to the loo. You can also take a tablespoon of soaked or ground linseed or a handful of prunes throughout the day to make sure you're not straining; fibre is your friend, as is staying well hydrated.

Not being able to control your wind after giving birth is common, as is leaking a little when you sneeze. But you should feel an improvement over time (see Chapter 15). Speak to your doctor if full control of your bladder or bowel does not return, because while this is a common problem, it should not become your new normal. They should refer you to a pelvic health physiotherapist, in line with NICE guidelines. You can also contact a physio directly: either refer yourself to an NHS practitioner (if self-referrals are possible in your area) or book a private appointment (see page 218, Getting Help). Even if you don't have symptoms, you may want to see a pelvic physiotherapist; experts warn that the pelvis is good at masking problems and compensating until later in life when symptoms creep in. These symptoms could be avoided by early ongoing rehab and an awareness of your bladder and bowel's health.

Anja describes the extraordinary recovery her body made within just a few weeks:
'My vagina was a bomb site and I couldn't predict where things would come from anymore, or even where to wipe. Just going for a wee was uncomfortable. The hospital had given me a squeezy bottle, which I used to stop the stinging. But I could feel my bladder pushing somehow on the front wall of my vagina, in a way that it never had done before, and I had no control if I coughed or sneezed. I remember exploring

my vagina in the shower – I just had no idea whether it was normal. As for having a poo – well, for a start it took ages to clean myself afterwards because I wasn't as defined as I used to be, and it was all quite tender. And then after I'd finished I had the indignity of needing to push my bottom back inside myself because it had sort of bulged out. I think it was a haemorrhoid. It was all deeply confusing but I didn't really know anything about prolapses, and just carried on. I did my pelvic floor exercises whenever I was breastfeeding and after a few weeks things seemed to be going back to normal. Well, I say normal, but it'll never feel like it used to – it's just different, but my essential functions now are largely back to how they were. It's extraordinary how the body recovers itself.'

Perineal irrigation

If you didn't get one at the hospital, you might like to treat yourself to a perineal irrigation bottle – a soft-sided bottle with a valve that you can squeeze water out of. You can buy a bottle that is designed for the job, order a squeezy sauce bottle like the sort used in professional kitchens (which are cheaper), or just try using a normal sports bottle. Use it whilst you wee, because urine irritates the broken skin if you've had any sort of tear or a cut down there. Warm water can also loosen uncomfortably tight stitches and keep the area clean to avoid infection. Fill the bottle and start squirting it onto yourself before you wee to dilute the urine. Continue until you're finished. You can also lean right forwards to direct the urine away from where it's sore. And, of course, you can resort to weeing in the shower. After washing, pat yourself dry with loo roll. People online extoll the benefits of using a hairdryer and claim that the heat helps with healing, but doctors don't recommend this as it can lead to tissue damage, even on a cold setting, and slow down healing.

Constipation

It's normal for your bowels to be a little confused for the first few weeks. Since everything will already be weak and a bit displaced, it's really important to avoid straining. Drink lots of water, eat high-fibre food (I've said it before, but linseed is brilliant) and, if necessary, take a stool softener or gentle laxative (see page 67). It helps to raise your feet on a small stool, bringing up your knees, whilst you go to the loo, or to lean forwards; flexing your hips beyond 90 degrees allows your bowels to work more easily. And, rather than hold your breath and push, take deep breaths into your tummy.

OASIs

OASIs (either third- or fourth-degree tears – see page 64) are the most common cause of faecal and flatus (or wind) incontinence in women – conditions that can occur independently, or together. A 2017 paper suggested that midwives and doctors miss about 40 per cent of these when they first inspect a woman's perineum after birth; sometimes they diagnose a second-degree tear instead and, not realising the anal sphincter is damaged, fail to repair it. The risk factors for OASIs include having a baby heavier than 4 kilograms (8.8 lbs), an instrumental delivery (especially forceps) and this being your first baby. OASIs can have serious consequences for the woman, such as faecal incontinence and severe pain, which can appear at any time, from immediately after the birth to much later in life. If you suspect there is any tear between your back passage and vagina that has not been diagnosed and repaired, speak to a healthcare professional to request an assessment. Symptoms include not being able to hold your bowels, having to rush to the loo because you need to open them and, in very rare cases, when stool or wind gets into your vagina.

Haemorrhoids

Also known as piles, haemorrhoids are bulging blood vessels like varicose veins that appear in your bum. If you avoided them during pregnancy, it's possible that one or more appeared during the birth due to the pressure on your abdomen and digestive system. They can form inside and outside of your body and can sometimes be pushed back inside if and when they appear. They can make wiping difficult – they can be very painful and it can feel like there's always more to clean – so wet wipes, wetting the toilet paper, or washing the area may help. If you're in pain or they're not going away on their own, see your doctor, who can prescribe a steroid cream that works quickly and can be used while breastfeeding.

> *Suzie's husband helped her to monitor her painful and persistent piles:*
> 'I got my husband to take a picture of my pile and vag wound to show me. At one point I thought it had burst as the pain suddenly decreased, just as the bleeding from my butt briefly exceeded that from my vagina. It bled for about three days whenever I did a poo. It's now stopped bleeding but an inspection last night showed it's still there. My husband's named him Percy. On a bad day, it's a really sharp pain,

but my vagina is hurting me more than my butt so it's hard to discern exactly what discomfort is coming from where. It doesn't help having to wrangle with a toddler as well – I keep thinking it's getting better then it gets worse again.'

12

Belly, Core and Floor

The sad fact of the matter is that giving birth doesn't necessarily stop you looking pregnant immediately. A few days after my son was born and I was starting to feel claustrophobic. No one had told me that you're meant to stay in bed – and certainly not meant to leave the house – for at least a week, so when we ran out of potatoes in the evening, I was quick to say I'd go to the shop. Too quick, in fact – I sounded desperate. 'I really don't mind going,' Philip insisted.

'No! I'll go.' The shop. Leaving the house on my own, with neither belly nor baby. As I sat behind the wheel of the car, I felt the improbable emptiness of my abdomen. At the local Spar, having taken longer than necessary to select some potatoes, I was marvelling at the array of tonic waters when a man I recognised from our local pub looked up from the beer shelf.

'Still not had it, then?' he said, looking down at my tummy.

I reddened at his non-question. 'No – I, er, have had it,' I said.

He didn't say anything to that; I think he was lost for words.

I shuffled off to the counter with my potatoes feeling humiliated. Having a belly and being pregnant is fine, but having the same belly and not being pregnant is not fine.

During pregnancy, the rectus abdominis muscles (the ones you see in a six-pack), that run vertically from your breast-bone to your pubic bone, move apart to accommodate the baby. After birth, they are long and weak, and the tissue that connects them has stretched, so you will feel a gap between them if you try to do a sit up. While your uterus starts con-tracting as soon as you've given birth, these muscles stay stretched and weak for a while longer. I remember thinking I could lose a car key inside my belly, so ample and doughy was the tissue. It's disconcerting, but your pre-pregnancy profile will come back with time. The key to regaining it lies in your posture, and your core, which includes your pelvic floor, diaphragm, abdominals and back muscles. To aid the process of rehabilitating your muscles and knitting them back together, you can make sure you eat and drink well, rest, gently increase your level of activity, and reconnect with your core using simple breathing exercises (see page 258).

Re-engaging your core

If you had a strong core before your pregnancy, you're likely to regain your strength more quickly than someone starting from scratch. But fear not – by gently increasing your level of activity, eating well and staying hydrated, you will help your body to recover at its own speed. For now, learn to reconnect with your abdominal muscles and pelvic floor; whether you had a physiological birth or a caesarean, they will be signifi-cantly weaker by now.

You'll notice that the below exercises (and almost all the core exercises referred to in this book) involve you contract-ing your muscles on or after your exhale, not when you inhale. This is because your core is essentially a pressurised cylinder, with the diaphragm on top, pelvic floor at the bottom, and muscles around the sides and up the front and back. When you breathe out, the cylinder's lid rises, reducing the pressure inside. This makes it easier for the other muscles – the pelvic floor and abdominals – to contract, as they encounter less resistance when they do so.

'The most vital and effective exercise you can do'

Wendy Powell of MUTU System advises that you do the following exercise as soon as you can after birth; you can even do it from bed at first. It is 'the most vital and effective exercise you can do,' she says.

Finding your pelvic floor and core muscles
Get comfortable and take a couple of deep breaths. Drop your shoulders. Drop your ribs. Inhale and let your abdominal muscles and pelvic floor relax. To find the right muscles, imagine you're trying really hard not to fart or wee, or that you're drawing a tampon up inside you. Exhale slowly as you lift and gently squeeze your pelvic floor. Your buttocks should stay relaxed. Breathe in again and relax. Don't push away or down, just let it all go as you inhale. Repeat the exhale and pelvic floor lift. You may feel your abdominal muscles drawing in or tensing as you engage your pelvic floor. This is good! The system is all connected and this tells you it is working. If you've had a caesarean, you may feel nothing in your abs for now, which is fine – some numbness and lack of sensation is normal. Repeat for five or six breaths. Take a moment to mindfully breathe through this exercise three times a day.

Protecting your abs

After birth, pretty much all women's abdominal muscles have
parted in order to make way for the baby inside your uterus,
and the connective tissue between them has stretched. The
muscles usually go back into place within a few months, but
while they're still parted, you'll notice that your belly domes
like a ridge line whenever you overload the muscles with
pressure, for example, when you try to sit up. You should
avoid causing the doming; it's a sign that the pressure in your
abdomen is overwhelming the muscles. But in the early days
you'll probably find that some doming is unavoidable; don't
beat yourself up when it happens, just try to maintain good
posture and modify how you do things to limit it.

Pelvic floor muscle training

Once you feel confident that everything is connected again
– your core, pelvic floor and the nerves that connect them
to your brain – you can move onto pelvic floor muscle training. This should include a combination of long pelvic floor
contractions to build strength for your everyday support,
and short, sharp contractions to improve your response to
things like sneezes and coughs. Once you master these, you
can build them into other exercises, like squats, or even make
them a part of your daily routine; for example, contract your
pelvic floor muscles whenever you're walking up the stairs
(see page 183).

Belly binding

For centuries, postnatal women have bound their tummies
with cloth to support the abdomen. It's believed to ease back

pain and strain on muscles and ligaments and to improve posture by holding the abdomen close to the spine, which is where it should be. In Malaysian culture, *bengkung* is the name for a length of fabric that traditionally wraps around the abdomen; in South America, they call it a *faja*, and in Japan, it's a *sarashi*. In Ayurvedic medicine, one of the oldest medical systems still in use today, belly binding is about more than just supporting your abdomen and putting your organs back where they came from. They believe that pregnancy creates an imbalance in the body – an excess of Vata, meaning space and air. Belly binding, according to Ayurveda, can stop you accumulating excess Vata after birth. Modern belly wraps – elastic and Velcro products – are becoming popular in an update of the bengkung tradition. They claim to minimise stretch marks and help to correct the separation of the abdominal muscles, as well as to shave inches from your waist, and provide support and reassurance; a modern-day corset.

However, the evidence for them is shaky and midwives in the UK don't usually recommend them. A 2013 study compared the effect of belly binding with daily abdominal exercises on a new mum's recovery. By the end of six weeks, all women had stronger abdominal muscles, and reduced waists and waist-to-hip ratios, but the women who'd done the exercises were in significantly better shape, with a reduced gap between their abdominal muscles, than those who'd worn the belly binds.

While belly binding isn't as effective as exercise when it comes to rebuilding abdominal strength, it can help with confidence, protect your caesarean scar, potentially reduce back and pelvic pain, and support you during activities. Just remember not to bind it too tight, because if you squeeze anything in the middle, things bulge out at the ends – and you certainly don't want that.

Rowena gave birth to her first baby by caesarean in a country where belly binding was routine, and wore a modern corset for weeks after the birth:
'We were living in Southeast Asia and I had an emergency C-section. Afterwards, the nurses just came and wrapped me in a corset. It really helped, particularly having that support over your scar. There's lots of advice that you should put your hand over the incision or hold a pillow to it when you cough or laugh, and I quickly realised that I didn't need that additional support. I had the feeling that it was pushing everything back together. It didn't irritate the stitches, because they had a big dressing over them, and the corset went over that. I did book a more traditional Indonesian tummy binding doula, who made me sit on a little chair over a hot pot of herbs. She was meant to wrap me in a proper Indonesian corset but it looked so painful. I politely declined and kept the modern, medical corset instead. I stopped wearing it when I was signed off by my doctor at six weeks. One of my friends from Brazil was horrified that I stopped wearing it so quickly. In Brazil, they wear them for months. When I had my second baby in the UK, a vaginal delivery, I tried to put it on myself but it just didn't feel right, and my midwife said they're not recommended here.'

How to try belly binding for yourself
In many cultures, binding kicks off with warm oils being massaged into the abdomen. After that, the cloth – or a more modern product that does the same job – is wrapped around

the belly and worn for anything from a few hours to a day or more at a time. The practice continues for anything up to six months, but more commonly four to six weeks. You can either buy one of the modern products available or, if you're feeling enterprising, make your own bengkung bind from a length of fabric about 14 metres long. Cut off a strip about eight inches wide, then turn to YouTube to learn how to tie it.

Annabel wore a modern belly bind after her caesarean whenever she wanted extra support:
'A lot of the time with a C-section you feel that you're going to pop a seam and everything is going to fall out. Having the support of that elasticated thing was so reassuring. I didn't use it for the first week or so because my stitches needed to heal – I started using it once the stitches felt fine. I wore it just for a few hours every day, whenever I was going to be active. For example, when I went out walking or when I was giving the baby a bath and knew that I'd be crouching down. It felt nice to have the support.'

13

Self-care

There will be times when just brushing your teeth and washing your face or having a shower will feel like a significant act of self-care. It was often the days when I felt most rotten that I would put more effort than usual into getting dressed, then add a lick of mascara or dig out a fancy serum that I hadn't used in months. You don't have to spend money to take care of yourself – just being mindful of what makes you feel good can help.

Massage

Thirty minutes of aromatherapy massage two days after birth can boost physical and mental health and even improve bonding with your baby, according to a 2006 study in the *Journal of Midwifery and Women's Health* – so if you are looking for an excuse to book a massage, there you go.

In many cultures, massage is a cornerstone of postnatal healing; it's common for women in Asia to receive a massage every day for up to a month postpartum. Massage claims to help with issues of breastmilk supply as it boosts oxytocin, which promotes milk flow; it releases tight muscles and encourages healing; it can improve sleep and energy levels; it can strengthen the immune system and relieve fluid retention; and it can regulate your hormones. If you've had a caesarean, practitioners recommend you hold off on massaging your abdomen until the scar has healed, but if you had a vaginal birth, you can include your abdomen from a week after the birth. Unfortunately, however, the West has done away with traditional healing practices during the postpartum phase and we regard having a massage therapist visit our homes as something of a luxury.

Tanya James, the massage and movement therapist behind Mother Massage in the UK, likes to see new mums for a massage as soon as possible. If you're massaging yourself, Tanya advises that you look for knots or painful spots in your body with your fingers and release them by applying gentle pressure. Applying pressure in strokes along the connective tissue in between your abdominal muscles can also improve skin tone and increase elasticity, helping to restore your muscle structure and stomach tone, she says. Use oils (or do it in the bath or shower) and make sure you're warm first.

Tanya believes massage can have a rapid and visible impact and showed me – a self-confessed cynic – pictures of her daughter's stomach before and after an abdominal massage, at about five weeks postpartum. In the 'after' picture, her stomach appears firmer, and the diastasis – the gap between the vertical abdominal muscles that part to make space for your baby – appears smaller. Is that really possible just through massage, I wonder?

Yes, it is, I'm later told – although it's not as simple as that. The body can change quickly as a result of massage, not just because the physical pressure impacts the tissue directly, but because it also works to recruit the brain and nervous system to the job of healing.

Olivia Inge, a London-based Chinese medical practitioner, acupuncturist and massage therapist, has spent nearly ten years exploring this philosophy, that you can stimulate the body's own healing process using holistic therapies like massage, acupuncture and aromatherapy. Before that, she spent years working as a catwalk model for the likes of Vivienne Westwood and Alexander McQueen. Despite being in possession of such an enviable body, she was no different to the rest of us in feeling reduced to a pair of boobs after childbirth. A week after her daughter was born, Olivia remembers a friend and yoga teacher appearing at her door like an angel to give her a massage; her friend noticed things about Olivia's body that she hadn't noticed herself, and that massage left her feeling whole again, and 'not just like a pair of tits that feed. She gave me that support, not only physically, but also emotionally,' Olivia said.

If you can get a massage at home, Olivia urges, do. Massage, she explains, tilts the brain's focus from stress towards relaxation and healing. It reduces naturally occurring biochemicals associated with depression; it changes your mood and promotes the physiological phenomena that encourage self-healing – unlocking the door to your internal pharmacy, as she says. You can also try to bring some of that healing energy into your everyday routines with simple self-care rituals that, even just for a few seconds, take you out of your head and into your body. Spend a little longer than necessary moisturising your face or washing your hair. Stretch. And breathe a little more deeply once in a while.

Olivia Inge recalls the power of her own postnatal massage:
'I didn't really feel like I was in my body after childbirth. I lost a lot of blood, which left me depleted; there was nothing

in the tank. It's vital that you keep the body–mind connection intact so you know when you have had enough of entertaining, need to sleep, or need to eat. You go through the motions, but you're just so knackered, and your world suddenly becomes consumed by this little thing that you've got to keep alive; your body is the tool. When a friend came to massage me about a week after the birth, it was exactly what I needed. If you're struggling with breastfeeding (which I was because my daughter had a tongue tie), you can start having miserable thoughts – why isn't this working? And then if you're not careful it's a domino effect and your thoughts start to affect your physiology. For the milk to come through, it's all just got to be right – and massage can help to regulate the hormones that you need. I remember my friend massaging my feet – it felt so good. She brought my awareness back to having a whole body again.'

Tips for self-care at home

There are some simple things that you can do at home to help you focus on yourself and take time out from your new baby.

Body brushing – Your lymph system is your body's drainage network, and since all of your organs have been working at maximum capacity during your pregnancy, powering hormone surges and crashes and moving 50 per cent more fluid around than usual, you'll find that there's a lot of excess fluid to get rid of. Brushing your body lightly all over – with just a little bit more pressure than a tickle – stimulates the lymph system that is running underneath the skin. As Olivia says, it's gentle, it's specific, and it feels good.

Mini head massage – When all that's running through your head is what you or the baby should or should not be doing, it can help to remind yourself that there's more to you than just a robotic cycle of feed, sleep, clean up, repeat. To take some of the energy away from your incessantly moving thoughts, run your hands through your hair and twist it, so you're gently pulling the skin on your scalp up. Then run your fingers around your scalp and neck and enjoy the moment of sensation. If you have a partner, it's even better to get them to do it.

Face massage – There are acupressure points all around your eyes – by the inside corners, the outside tips of your brows, and directly under the eye between the fleshy bit and bone. Using your index finger, scoop underneath from the inside corner to the outer edge, fall into your temples and press three times, then move down where the ear joins the face and a bunch of lymph nodes sit. Then sweep under your cheekbones with as much pressure as you can muster – a lot of energy gets stuck here – up to your nostrils, then down your smile lines to your jaw, then sweep under the jawline from the middle to the outside edges of your jaw. You can then sweep down your neck from your windpipe out to the sides of your neck. This helps to drain excess fluid as well as toxins from your face.

Foot bath – Soak your feet in warm water with a few drops of pure lavender oil; it's another little act of self-care that helps pull excess energy away from your exhausted mind and redirects it to your feet and out of your body.

Follow the energy lines – While lying in the bath (or using oil), start with your fingers at the outside edge of your little toe, where your bladder meridian (one of your twelve energy lines, according to Chinese medicine) ends. Using long strokes, sweep up your leg and the front of your body up to your neck, and then down your forearms to your fingertips. Then come back again along the underside of your arm, up to your armpit and down the side of your body, back down the backs of your legs and ending again at the little toe.

Tennis ball massage – If you have particular sore spots or a bad back, another way of massaging yourself is by using a tennis ball or two. If you have lower back pain, place two tennis balls inside a sock, knot the end, and lie on top of it so that one ball is either side of your spine. Move your body up and down the balls until you find a tight spot that needs releasing, relax and lie into it until you feel the pain dissipate. Move it slightly, then try again. You can also massage your bum, which is often linked to back problems, and your feet like this.

14

The Six-week Check

In an online survey, the postnatal fitness gurus behind MUTU System, an online exercise programme designed for new mums and one of the few apps that NHS Digital recommends, asked women what they had googled rather than asked a medical professional after childbirth. 'Everything,' was one of the most common answers. I consider myself good at asking questions; I'm a journalist, and I spend my life talking about difficult subjects. It therefore baffles me that I was the same, and did not ask any of the questions I wanted answers to at my six-week check-up. As the Irish writer Anne Enright puts it, 'I draw upon however many ghastly generations of suffering have preceded me and say that everything is fine, wonderful, marvellous.' Saying that I was well was partly true: I was falling in love with my baby and felt deeply happy. But I was also unstable, anxious, leaky, misshapen, adrift, and occasionally scared.

I got the notoriously brusque nurse, who skimmed over the basics quickly. She took my blood pressure, then asked about feeding.

'No pain when you pass urine or solids?'

'No.' (Honest answer.)

She didn't ask whether I leaked or could control my wind, so I ventured no information on the matter. I would have liked her to ask. But what I really wanted was for her to look between my legs and add some weight to my husband's hypothesis that everything was OK. Why did she not offer? Did she not have any idea how unsure I might be feeling, or how difficult it can be to ask a stranger to look at your vagina? One friend told me she almost had to beg her doctor to examine her, such was the doctor's reluctance. If there was ever a next time, I remember thinking, I'd be more forthright.

Before my less-than-illuminating six-week check came to a close, the nurse said, 'So, no postnatal depression?' It was her offhand manner that surprised me most. Would I really say 'yes' at this point, if I did have postnatal depression? Suddenly I wanted to cry, though, so maybe her question was spot on. But no, she had no time for tears; before I knew it, I was out of the door. And that was it, my sole opportunity to share with a healthcare professional the many daunting, niggling and disquieting things affecting me and my body – and I hadn't mentioned any of them, because she hadn't asked, and I'd been too shell-shocked to enquire.

What is the six-week check?

Traditionally, women have always seen a GP at six weeks postpartum, where they are checked and – hopefully – signed off for exercise and sex. In recent years, this check-up has included screening for postnatal depression. Despite improvements, these appointments remain controversial. Physiotherapists argue that the notion of a six-week sign-off is not appropriate; a woman's body (especially her pelvis and pelvic organs) take far longer than six weeks to fully recover. GPs with an interest in postpartum health lament the fact that they get so little time for such an important and complex task – the standard ten minutes, they say, is barely enough to cover the basics, let alone to examine a woman to see how she's healing and get a sense of her mental health. Other GPs consider them 'a worthless, unscientific tradition' and relic of 'the dark ages', as one recently wrote in the GP magazine, *Pulse*; postpartum women should see their doctor when they have a problem, not universally and arbitrarily at six weeks. And women themselves often describe these appointments as a complete waste of time. They are rarely made to feel like they can truly talk about their concerns, in part because of time constraints, and also because of the taboo that shrouds common issues like incontinence, pain in the vagina or perineum, and wind. Nearly half of new mothers' mental health problems are missed by health professionals at the six-week check, according to a recent study by the UK charity, the National Childbirth Trust.

And even when women do talk openly with their GP, their symptoms are often dismissed as 'normal'. Even though early intervention is considered key when it comes to pelvic health, women are regularly told to wait and see after presenting with clear symptoms of prolapses, anal sphincter damage or pelvic floor dysfunction. Your symptoms should never be dismissed as normal, but too many GPs don't have the training to understand them, and too many NHS trusts don't have the budgets they need to address them. As a result, women like Ella (see Chapter 15 on the pelvic floor) live for months, sometimes years, with their problems getting worse because their GPs can't give them the advice or the referral that they need. Don't be afraid to insist on a follow-up appointment and to stand up to get what you want and need.

If you know the shortcomings of our system and decide in advance what you want to get out of your six-week check, it can, however, be a valuable opportunity to seek advice and help, so make the best of it. I wish I had.

> *Clare Bourne, pelvic health physiotherapist, on what is often the reality of the six-week check:*
> 'At the six- to eight-week check, if this is available in your area, a large part of your GP's focus is on mental health, which is important, but if a woman has physical symptoms of pelvic floor dysfunction this is a really important time for it to be picked up; the earlier they receive help the better and we know that pelvic floor dysfunction has an impact on mental health, so really they go hand in hand. Women view this check as a sign-off for exercise, however, without a thorough physical examination it is not possible to do this, and unless a woman is symptomatic, referral is not possible on the NHS for physiotherapy at the moment.

How to get the most out of your six-week check

I interviewed a number of GPs with a particular interest in women's health, and drew from their insights the following advice:

- If you want to discuss something sensitive or complicated, request a double appointment so you can take your time.
- Consider explaining to the receptionist that you would like their most understanding doctor to talk about a personal physical (or mental) problem.
- Doctors and nurses see bottoms and vaginas every day – while you may find it embarrassing, it's just part of their routine.

- People find it hard to admit they're struggling; you don't need to name a problem if you find it difficult, just try to start a conversation so your doctor can, at least, book a follow-up appointment to look out for you.
- If you're not offered a six-week check, as you should be, ask for one – it's important; and ask to see the GP who specialises in women's health.
- Doctors don't usually ask specifically about bowel control, something women can find very embarrassing, but they do want to know about it. If you have any concerns, try to bring them up so that they can help you.
- If you feel uncomfortable describing your problem, find words that make it easier – for example, say your bladder isn't quite right, so your doctor can broach the subject gently.
- Book a follow-up appointment at three months postpartum if there's anything you're unsure of – you can cancel it if the issue resolves but, if it doesn't, there's a fair chance you'll need help to solve it; 92 per cent of those who are incontinent at 12 weeks, for example, will still be incontinent at five years, according to one recent study.

Dr Fiona Brodie-Fraser, GP and mother of three, describes how she conducts a six-week check:
'It's most important that women feel comfortable attending their appointment, so I'm always trying to put them at ease. We usually do a double booking of 20 minutes. I normally start by asking a few general questions: are you feeling happy in yourself, how is the feeding going, how are things at

home? One of the questions is, are you enjoying your baby? I think that's a really useful question for flagging up any depression. Some women will say, yes – it's lovely. Others will say it's really hard work but they're happy. And there are some women who say, I'm just exhausted. We talk about how they're coping, what kind of support they're getting, and hopefully I give them the opportunity to say, I'm finding this really hard. We talk about what the options are, including increased health visitor support. Depending on how low they're feeling and what their past experiences are, they might need medication, but probably, if it's mild, it will just be extra support and follow-up appointments so they can talk it through again. It can be nice to know that your GP has children, and male GPs can be just as understanding because they've also done the sleepless nights and had screaming babies.

'In practical terms, I make sure the baby has had its hearing check, ask about the baby, how the mother's breasts are feeling, and, if they're not breastfeeding, whether their breasts have settled down. I'll ask what's happening with the bleed – it should pretty much have stopped by this time. And I'll ask if they've had a period yet, and talk about contraception. Some people look at me like I'm mad to even suggest it, and other people will say, well, actually we've been using condoms. There's a huge range, from those talking about getting pregnant already to those who aren't going to be ready for a sexual relationship until the baby is six months old because they're exhausted and there are other things on their mind. Either end of the spectrum is fine, as long as both partners are happy. I would need to check blood pressure and weight if they decide to start on oral contraceptives.

'After that, I will offer an examination. If everything is

comfortable and they don't want an examination, that's fine. But if they're worried that it's still sore or doesn't feel right, or they've tried intercourse and it was painful – if they've got any concerns at all – then I do a vaginal examination. If they've had a caesarean, I offer to look at the scar to make sure it's OK. Then I check blood pressure, and weight, although that might not be anything like back to normal.

'If a woman has symptoms of prolapse then I would make sure we talk through pelvic floor exercises and there'd be a referral to the gynae-physios at the local hospital, where they'd get a course of sessions. Usually, that will be enough. Likewise, bladder and bowel problems. There are also sometimes problems post-episiotomy; scar tissue can be uncomfortable with intercourse. Sometimes things settle down or you can manually relax it, but some people just scar more easily than others and end up with tissue that's very tight and doesn't stretch easily. If it's still really uncomfortable at two or three months, we refer back to the gynaecologists. You shouldn't be suffering with painful intercourse if you've had an episiotomy or a tear repaired – you should be able to get something done about that.'

Part 3

STRONGER IN THE LONG RUN

When asked what I do, I define myself in two ways: as a writer, and a runner. The two are linked – some of my best work has come out of running; it's when I decompress and ask questions of myself. I don't always enjoy these activities – both writing and running have a unique capacity to make me feel anxious, guilty and filled with self-doubt, especially for not doing them – but I suspect that somewhere therein lies the reason I keep coming back to them. It took me a few decades to work this out and, by the time I had my baby, shortly before my 35th birthday, I knew that writing and running were the two things I did. I thought that was the end of the story. Having my baby, however, took both of them away from me. Suddenly, I had no time or energy to write, and I lacked the strength I needed to run; sometimes, it felt like I was just sitting at home breastfeeding while my identity drifted away out of the window.

A number of women have said to me that it's not being a mum that's difficult, but not being yourself anymore. That's why swimming in the river that flows from the mountains of Snowdonia through the valley below our house helped me more than anything else. It took just minutes and, even if I felt completely sapped beforehand, left me feeling outrageously alive. When our baby was almost six months old, I remember barely flinching at the shock as I half jumped, half dived, into the swollen river from a muddy bank. It was spring and the sun had broken through the clouds. I swelled with pride as liquid ecstasy made me untouchable to the cold.

Feeling yourself is not easy when your body is still bearing the repercussions of birth. In my case, the problem was my pelvic floor muscles. For other women, it can be anxiety that drains them of their life-force. For others, it can be physical pain. And, as with sleep deprivation, it's only when things get back to normal – or something gets so bad you can't ignore it – that you start to see how much something has affected you.

We've all heard a version of the line, *what's best for the baby is whatever's best for you.* Yet we persistently subordinate our own needs to those of our baby. Pelvic health experts would like to see all women who've given birth around 12 weeks afterwards – the optimum time for addressing problems – but, unless symptoms are really chronic, this rarely happens because we are all too wrapped up in caring for our babies at that point, and even if your GP does refer you for physiotherapy, a first appointment can take months to materialise.

Statistics back up the fact that too many of us are suffering problems in silence. Roughly a quarter of new mums still find sex painful a year and a half after giving birth, according to studies, and only a fraction of them seek help. Half still have urinary incontinence, and more than three-quarters complain of back pain a year later. The barriers to us getting help are many and various, from the fact that access to specialist care on the NHS can be a postcode lottery, to being too busy and exhausted to tackle it ourselves. Treatment pathways are haphazard. And, if you do make it to your GP, you may – like I did – find that they normalise whatever problem you have. I've seen specialists leap out of their chairs with frustration when I relayed the story of my GP telling me that 'a degree of incontinence and prolapse is normal after childbirth and should get better with time'.

The problems women experience postpartum – like painful sex, leaky bladders or back pain – are common, but should not be accepted as a new normal; if they haven't gone away by around 12 weeks, we should be treating them, not living with them. This means, unfortunately, that it falls on us as women to demand more – more support, more appointments, more understanding, more recognition and more honesty. The goal of this section is to equip you with what you need to make informed choices about your mind and body in the year or two after having a baby, but also beyond, such as when pelvic floor problems arise later in life.

Postnatal fitness is, some physiotherapists argue, wrapped up in a culture of fear, where women are constantly told they mustn't do things – such as lift anything heavier than their baby, do a plank, drink coffee (if they're breastfeeding), run – and are made to feel fragile and weak. The blanket advice, to check with a physiotherapist before you do just about anything, is also problematic, because physiotherapy is often only available to those with the money to pay for it. I hope the information in this section empowers you to make better choices about your health, because it is *your* body. If you listen to it and something doesn't feel right, experts urge, stop doing it and seek help. But that doesn't mean you shouldn't feel strong – you are strong in uncountable ways.

15

Pelvic Floor – Incontinence, Prolapse and Pain

This is the first and lengthiest chapter in this section because the pelvic floor is at the root of the most common and debilitating (not to mention taboo) issues affecting women in the long term – urinary incontinence, bowel problems, pain in the pelvic area and prolapse. We'll look at the conditions individually, and how to treat them, but first I'll tell my story and then help you to understand the pelvic floor, one of the most underrated structures in the body.

My story

A few months after the birth, Philip and I were walking a friend's dogs through some woods. He carried the baby and I had the dogs on long leads so they could run around. When the terrier spotted something in one direction and the Labrador something in another, they propelled me forwards and wrapped me around the trunk of a tree. Arms akimbo, giggling helplessly, the inevitable mini wee occurred. I later heard someone say that women have a particular talent for experiencing joy and sorrow simultaneously. Indeed, they are right. But, as bittersweet as it was to wet my pants laughing, it wasn't something I intended to keep on doing.

For months, I squeezed my pelvic floor whenever I breast-fed – but it didn't seem to make any difference. Approaching six months, I joined the four-week waiting list to see my GP. I wanted to run again – I needed to run again – but I still couldn't even jog without my pelvic floor bouncing around like a trampoline. The doctor was female and a mother but in spite of this looked mildly inconvenienced when I asked her to examine me. After a brief look, she told me that eve-rything was as she'd expect and that it was normal to have a degree of incontinence and prolapse after birth. She glossed over my request for physiotherapy, instead giving me an A4 printout that dictated I do more squeezes each day. She said it should get better with time and that, even if it didn't, she wouldn't propose treatment until I'd completed my family, because subsequent births can do more damage.

I was initially relieved; who doesn't want a normal vagina? In time, however, I came to see her words as absurd. Just three years before, I'd been sickened by the inequality that left mothers in Africa leaking, as a result of fistulas from childbirth, for the rest of their lives. And now, here I was, accepting incontinence because it was 'normal'.

Giving up on the NHS, I contacted a pelvic health physio-therapist who charged £80 for an hour's session – a price worth paying, if I came away knowing what was going on and what I needed to do. Unfortunately, however, my recov-ery story is more a catalogue of errors than an exemplary guide. My continence got worse before it truly got better, and it was not time but knowledge and hard work that eventually made it come right.

The physiotherapist was dour and academic, and began with a long list of very detailed, very personal, questions.

As well as leaking, I was going to the loo more than once a night, and I didn't seem able to empty my bladder properly. I then lay down, and she put her finger inside me and gave instructions: 'Tense, release, tense and tell me when you release, tense as hard as you can ...' She rated my pelvic floor strength a miserable two out of a possible five; more than a mere flicker but very much sub-par.

She told me that I shouldn't expect my body ever to be the same again – which was not what I wanted to hear – then gave me homework, which involved giving up caffeine and keeping a urine diary, measuring and recording every millilitre of fluid in and out, for three days. Those in the throes of early motherhood will understand how impossible that sounded. I'm not usually a quitter, and I hate wasting money, but I aborted the bladder diary after finding it unworkable, whilst in sole charge of a six-month-old, to measure and record the volume of my drinks and wee for three days. As for giving up caffeine, I considered moving to France, where they have free pelvic floor physiotherapy and a healthy respect for espresso.

Feeling sheepish – because I also knew that she was probably right – I never contacted the physio again. Instead, I carried on, feeling let down, until – as the GP promised – time did its work and I could just about keep up with my toddler as he ran through fields of buttercups. And as my ability to run returned incrementally, I felt the last of the grey clouds clear from above my head. I thought that was it; my recovery would be a linear thing, and the worst was over. But I was wrong. The following winter, shortly after my baby turned two, three things happened almost simultaneously: I signed the contract for this book, got an awful cough that persisted for about a month, and experienced an alarming regression – I could no longer hold my bladder. I then discovered I was pregnant.

I do not recommend conducting a research project into all of the things that can befall a woman's body after pregnancy whilst actually being pregnant yourself – but, if you do, it certainly injects a sense of gravity and imperative into your work. I have now interviewed countless pelvic health experts, but it was an interview with the esteemed Dr John DeLancey, the Norman F. Miller Professor of Gynecology at the University of Michigan, that made things fall into place. I first came across John in an article published by the American magazine *Mother Jones*. The article quoted John as saying that Kegel exercises, as recommended to strengthen a woman's pelvic muscles, do not appear to help. 'It's what everyone would like to believe,' John says, 'but I don't think there's any evidence to support it.'

I reread the paragraph to check I hadn't misunderstood anything, but no, it seemed clear; the grandfather of modern pelvic floor health was saying that doing pelvic floor squeezes, in the way that the NHS recommends, doesn't work. And I'd spend the last two and a half years doing them. How on earth have so many people, including our beloved health service, got it so wrong?

I emailed John immediately to better understand this and, to my surprise, received a call a few hours later. John, who has specialised in women's pelvic floor health for some 30 years, leads a multidisciplinary team including biomechanical engineers, nurse researchers, public health experts, practising doctors and physiotherapists, and has received some $25 million of US government grants to establish sound evidence for what works and what doesn't when it comes to pelvic health. This man, with his disarmingly kind and patient manner, is as high an authority as you can get. And he had a personal stake in the matter; his daughter-in-law was about to give birth. As I'd expected, he told me that it's not quite as simple as the *Mother Jones* article made out. But it's true that doing Kegels in the watered-down way that some media articles prescribe today does not help with stress incontinence, for example, when you sneeze. Rehabilitating a muscle needs targeted, high-intensity work. The NHS telling us all to squeeze three times a day is like treating an infection with a tenth of the effective dose, John said, or like a weight-lifter trying to increase their strength by lifting 500 grams.

So, what should we be doing to strengthen a damaged pelvic floor? John told me about a leading expert in pelvic floor training, Kari Bø, in Norway, whose work shows that it takes about 20 minutes of intensive pelvic floor and core exercises three times a week to improve symptoms. According to Kari's proven regimen, pelvic floor exercises need to be done at or close to maximum intensity, under regular supervision, for at least eight weeks; the more intensive the better. I later learned that, if the muscles aren't damaged, you can then progress to loading them while you train them by doing squats or lifting weights, or doing the exercises while you're doing something else, such as climbing the stairs; then you'll really start to see a difference. Why did no one tell me this?

John's smooth, confident voice then dropped another bombshell: there is a much simpler treatment for bladder control that is proven to be effective, which is skill training, as opposed to muscle strengthening – something I'd never even heard of before. The simple act of learning skills and techniques to control your bladder can cut incontinence by half, according to John's colleague Dr Janis Miller's research (see page 237). After I thanked John for his time and hung up, I spent half an hour browsing an interactive website about bladder training, created by Dr. Miller, that John had mentioned: myconfidentbladder.org. The information it contained was revolutionary and, within a few nights, I was sleeping for the first time in nearly three years without getting up to use the loo – and all for free!

What is the pelvic floor?

Your core muscles include the diaphragm, back muscles, abdominal muscles and pelvic floor; they form the roof, walls and floor of your abdomen – like a house. Together, these muscles are responsible for posture, balance, continence and stability, while your pelvic floor also supports your bladder, bowel and womb. The pelvic floor muscles are attached to your pubic bone at the front and your tailbone at the back, and your pelvic organs rest on them like a hammock. It is one of the hardest-working muscle groups in the body, constantly interacting with your different parts as you move around.

The openings for each organ – the urethra from the bladder, the rectum from the bowel and the vagina from the uterus – pass through gaps in the muscle to allow your body to dispose of water and waste, and for sex and reproduction to take place. People refer to their functions as 'the three Ss': supportive, sphincteric and sexual. In addition to their supporting role, they allow us to prevent leaks and squeeze out the last of our wee or poo, and, in women, they tighten the vagina, maintain clitoral erections when you're aroused and contract rhythmically when you orgasm. But they can become weak and their functions compromised; the biggest causes of weakness are pregnancy, obesity and ageing. There are three layers to your pelvic floor. It's the deepest layer,

STRONG PELVIC FLOOR

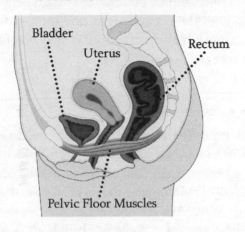

which includes a muscle known as the *levator ani*, which is attached at the front and back of the pelvis, that can become partly detached from the pubic bone during childbirth, and the top layer, including the superficial perineal muscles, that often tears.

Because the core muscles often work together, you'll find that many exercises for the pelvic floor strengthen other muscles in the core in tandem. If you find that you engage your deep abdominal muscles at the same time as your pelvic floor, this is good – there is a synergy between the two, and strengthening one can help the other.

If you ever did athletics at school, you may recall learning that we all have both fast- and slow-twitch muscle fibres; the general rule is that fast-twitch fibres are good for bursts of energy like sprinting, and slow-twitch fibres are better suited to endurance races. The muscles of your pelvic floor are no different, and you need to train both types of muscle in order to maintain your conformation and continence. Like the difference between long-distance running and sprinting, the slow-twitch fibres do the endurance work, keeping us continent throughout the day and night, and the fast-twitch fibres act when a powerful contraction is needed, for example, when you sneeze.

Pelvic floor dysfunction

The goings-on inside your pelvis cannot be viewed in isolation in order to be understood. Research links incontinence to having a gap between your abdominal muscles, for example, and physical pain in your pelvis is often linked to mental pain in your mind. And it even works vice-versa, as problems in your pelvis can cause problems elsewhere. It took a friend of mine two years and four different therapists to work out that the cause of the pain in her shoulder was – you guessed it – all the way down in her pelvis. Despite this interplay and overlap, it's helpful to understand the commonest pelvic problems individually, including urinary incontinence, bowel problems including constipation and incontinence, pelvic pain and prolapses.

Pelvic muscle tone

Pelvic floor problems largely fall into this category: either the muscles are too tense (overall, or in specific areas), or too weak. Pregnancy and childbirth commonly weaken the pelvic floor muscles, thanks to the extra weight you carry around, the slackening effect of hormones and, if you go into labour, the contractions and eye-watering stretch they need to achieve to let the baby through. They stretch to up to four times their original length and may not be strong enough afterwards to close off your bladder and bowel when you need them to. Similarly, they might not be strong enough to stop you taking in air or water. If you have a bath after giving birth, don't be surprised if, when you stand up, water suddenly gushes out. One woman I interviewed described how, years after her births, 'I still get out of swimming pools and find I've taken half of the water with me.'

At the other end of the spectrum, the tissue can also become tight in places, and the muscles too tense to relax – and relaxation is vital for pain-free loo breaks and sex. This can happen as a result of physical damage such as tears, but also stress, fear, trauma or pain – or even clenching the muscles for too long, for example, if you work out a lot at the gym. Imagine a nervous puppy with its tail between its legs. Like ours, a dog's pelvic floor muscles are connected by neural pathways to its emotions, and are responsible for it wagging when happy and clamping down when uncomfortable or anxious.

Bladder behaviour

Another problem is that your bladder, which is also made of muscle, can go a bit haywire. It's common to develop an over-active bladder during pregnancy – like a needy puppy, it can be constantly demanding that you go to the loo, including at night, or give you a sudden and uncontrollable urge to wee. By being firm with it and saying 'no' when it decides it needs to empty for the third time in as many hours, you can calm it down and, eventually, stop the urge to go (see page 191).

Tissue damage

If you had any sort of cut or tear during childbirth, you may find your scar tissue is tight and painful; massaging the scar can help to relax the tissue, something a pelvic health physio-therapist can help you to do. In some women, the scar tissue is particularly problematic and difficult to release, in which case you'll need a gynaecologist or pelvic health physiothera-pist to help.

Avulsion and prolapse

In the nineties, John DeLancey discovered a new injury that has revolutionised our understanding of postpartum pelvic health. In childbirth, the deep muscle of the pelvic floor, the levator ani, can become detached from the pubic bone – like the tent I described in Chapter 2, where one or both of the guy ropes at the front becomes severed; the tent still stays up, but it's structurally less sound. Known as a levator ani muscle avulsion, it happens in 10 to 30 per cent of vagi-nal births, and can be the leading cause of prolapse over a woman's lifetime.

Physiotherapists describe it as their 'oh-my-God' moment, when they realised that it wasn't nerve damage making certain patients difficult to treat, but the fact that their key muscle had actually detached from the pelvis. Often, forceps are the cause; you're three times more likely to end up with an avulsion after a forceps delivery than after a ventouse cap. Big babies like mine and a mother's age are also risk factors.

There is no cure; the muscle doesn't reattach itself to bone, and surgical options aren't great. Before you panic as I did, however, remember that the pelvic floor muscles are attached at the back as well and only one part of the muscle is affected. An avulsion only leaves them partially detached; with training, the back will learn to compensate for the front.

Medical professionals aren't sure there's a need to diagnose an avulsion, although a good physio can usually feel that a part of the muscle is missing. It gives you a higher-than-average risk of prolapse as you go through life, and sometimes symptoms don't appear for 30 years or more, so if knowing about it might motivate you to work on your muscle strength and stability, then it's likely a good thing. If you suspect you do have an avulsion, the best course of action to prevent a prolapse in the future is to keep your BMI down and pelvic floor strength up.

Nerve damage

The pudendal nerve is the most important nerve in your pelvis; it runs through the lower back and branches out into the perineum, pelvic organs, urethra, vagina and rectum, where it is responsible for sensation and control. It gets squashed and damaged in over 30 per cent of vaginal deliveries, most commonly during the second stage of labour, and particularly if you're actively pushing for a long time. Usually symptoms get better with time, but about one in five women will still be symptomatic at six weeks and need treatment. Symptoms include wind and faecal incontinence, urinary incontinence, perineal pain, loss of sensation and problems with sex (see page 201).

Second babies and beyond

As I was writing this book, my second baby was growing slowly inside me. At first, I was able to draw a line between my work and the little person who would soon need to find his or her way out of me. After five months of writing about the adverse consequences of birth, however, I would spend low moments considering a private caesarean: I envisaged apocalyptic scenes, where either my pelvic floor would open up into a gaping cavern as the second baby – likely to be even bigger than my first – descended, or where my organs would drop down like a dairy cow's udders, their support structure having already been cut loose. In more lucid moments, I recognised that these eventualities were unlikely – but I was nevertheless relieved to discover a study in the *Journal of Obstetrics and Gynaecology* that found it's usually just the first birth that does the most damage to the pelvic floor structure; subsequent births tend to have less effect, and a second vaginal birth without forceps doesn't seem to cause any more damage to your deep musculature at all.

Urinary incontinence

The first thing you need to do if you have problems with urinary incontinence is identify your triggers. Is it something like sneezing? If so, see page 239 for information on stress incontinence. Do you need a wee whenever you enter the house, or do you get up multiple times in the night? If so, see page 191 for information on urge incontinence. Often, it's a combination of these things, in which case you need to address each separately. (Even if you have neither of these problems immediately after the birth, it's worth keeping your pelvic floor in shape – see page 179 – because 30 per cent of women who are continent to start with after birth develop symptoms within seven years.)

Stress incontinence – When you sneeze, do you cross your legs? Might you leak on a trampoline? If yes, then you have some stress incontinence. Stress urinary incontinence is the involuntary leakage of urine because of increased intra-abdominal pressure. You can usually fix it by learning to connect with the right pelvic floor muscles, teaching your body to tense them at the right time, and then strengthening them through pelvic floor muscle training (see page 200 for more).

Urgency and frequency – Do you ever go from having no urge to wee to suddenly needing to desperately? If yes, you likely have some 'urgency'. If it gets to the point where you actually leak, it becomes 'urge incontinence'. Alternatively, you may just find you need to go for a wee more often than normal (which is thought to be a maximum or six or seven times per day). Known as frequency, this happens when your body tells you it needs a wee when, physically speaking, it could easily hold on – sometimes for hours. If you're also getting up more than twice in the night to wee – a condition known as nocturia – then it's likely you have an overactive bladder, which is a combination of these things (urgency/urge incontinence, nocturia and frequency).

Whatever your issue, it's likely that your bladder – and not your pelvic floor – is the culprit. The bladder is a muscle and, just like any muscle, it can get twitchy and communication can go awry. The nerves that tell the brain the bladder needs to empty can also get damaged, resulting in inaccurate signalling. You can usually fix these problems by learning about your condition and making simple changes to your behaviour (see page 237).

Mixed urinary incontinence – The most common sort of urinary incontinence, this includes a bit of both stress and urgency.

Incontinence products and the normality trap

In a 2019 advert for TENA incontinence pads, a beautiful young mother pulls on a pair of black knickers while her baby sleeps in a cot next to her. 'I knew being a mum would have a few surprises. Nobody mentioned incontinence though,' she says to the camera. At this point the camera focuses on her knickers for the big reveal – they're not black knickers at all, but incontinence pants. She then pulls on a pair of tight-fitting jeans. 'A little bit of wee is not going to stop me being me,' she adds, giving a cute but defiant look to the camera. Soon after its release, the Royal College of Nursing denounced the ad for inaccurately portraying that 'it is normal to be incontinent post childbirth'.

In another TENA advert, seven fit-looking women (mums, we assume) are in skimpy gym gear doing an intense trampoline workout class. As they jump in time to the music, legs splayed, they say together, seemingly with euphoria, 'I – just – had – an – "oops" – moment.' It's the same message as the last ad – that leaking doesn't matter, it isn't going to stop you being yourself – and ingenious marketing. While it appears to be empowering women, it is doing the opposite by normalising a remediable health problem and encouraging reliance on an expensive and unnecessary product; neither advert mentions the fact that incontinence can be treated.

Sales of incontinence pads are skyrocketing. Forma-care, who make adult incontinence pads and pull-up pants, say the British market for their products, currently worth £300 million, is growing 'exponentially' and will almost double in the next decade. It is, on the one hand, great that women have the option of buying slimline disposable incontinence pants should they want them, or of joining a trampoline workout class; who doesn't like trampolining? The trouble is that we're losing sight of what's normal, thanks to the influence of profit-making organisations, and being channelled into making poor decisions for our health. Incontinence is common, but not 'normal' or inevitable; if you have symptoms, you should not ignore them. You certainly shouldn't do an intense trampolining workout; physiotherapists recommend that you stop doing an exercise before it brings on symptoms in order to do it safely.

The UK's health watchdog NICE agrees. Women should not routinely manage their symptoms using pads, she-pees (funnels that help you wee while out and about), or any other incontinence product, they say, because they're not going to help in the long run and may mean you just defer the problem. Instead, NICE recommends at least three months of supervised pelvic-floor muscle training as the first-line treatment; use incontinence pads to cope in the run-up to treatment or alongside ongoing therapy, and only use them in the long term if you have explored every other option. So, if you're buying incontinence pads but haven't seen a pelvic health physiotherapist yet, stop and think about treating the problem, not the symptom. If you can't get an NHS physio, consider the fact that you may be able to stop the leaking for good by following the exercises prescribed by a physio; one private appointment might cost the same as ten packs of TENA's incontinence pants – and could one day mean you don't wind up in a nursing home.

Bowel problems

Of all the myriad things that women can experience after giving birth, problems relating to their bowels are often among the most sensitive and taboo. It's not something we talk about before giving birth but a significant proportion of women will have trouble controlling gas or solids after a vaginal delivery. At one end of the spectrum, this can be fairly harmless. I once raised the question of postpartum wind in a WhatsApp group of six mums, and each chimed in with her own amusing tale of accidental farting after birth. At the other end of the spectrum, third- or fourth-degree tears can lead to a lifetime of physical and psychological issues that will never truly be resolved. If something feels wrong with you, it's important that you overcome any natural reluctance to talk about your bottom and find the words that will allow you to access help.

Constipation

We are all told to be careful lifting heavy objects after birth, but how many of us consider the effect of regularly bearing down to poo? If you often have to push to go to the loo, adjust your diet and/or fluid intake (see page 67). It took me two and a half years to discover ground linseed and, six months later, I'm still buying the stuff; just a tablespoon a day, as Mary Poppins might say. Remember also to raise your feet or bend your upper body forwards whilst you poo. If you're struggling to solve your constipation, however, the answer could lie elsewhere; it could be a symptom of a rectal prolapse, for example, and a good pelvic health physio should be able to help you get to the bottom of it.

Bowel incontinence

Damage to the anal sphincter during childbirth is common – studies of ultrasounds suggest defects occur in between

20 and 35 per cent of women after a vaginal birth – and can result in wind or faecal incontinence. The damage isn't always symptomatic at first, and incontinence rates are higher amongst mums diagnosed with OASIs (see page 64), which occur in about 10 per cent of vaginal births. If injuries to the muscles around the anus are identified and skilfully repaired at birth, they shouldn't cause you long-term problems. If, however, they aren't identified, or aren't repaired well, the injuries may leave you unable to control wind or stools, or you may have to rush to the loo as you cannot wait (known as urgency).

Women on the pain of bowel incontinence:
'I prefer to keep it a secret.'
'I'm afraid to go out of the house.'
'Apart from being very anxious, stressed and emotionally drained, I find my condition degrading.'
'We have not had any sexual encounters since the birth over three years ago.'
'I have no control of wind, which is a great embarrassment.'
'I do not feel attractive; it strips away your femininity.'
'Nobody warned me about this.'

Ending the stigma

It was Professor Mike Keighley, a retired colorectal surgeon who lives in the Midlands, who made me think differently about OASIs and faecal incontinence. Mike is passionate about everything he does, whether it's his watercolours of North Wales or his charity, the MASIC Foundation, which aims to lower rates of serious birth injuries and help new mums who are suffering in silence. Mike retired early, in part because of his outspokenness in criticising NHS services. His desire to help people and his natural curiosity led him to India, where he set up a bowel surgery unit in a large hospital. There, he got to know women without full bowel control, and discovered just how much it impacts them. 'They were in a really black place, psychologically,' he said, 'battling guilt, isolation, crashing self-confidence and the desire to hide their condition.' He was so moved by the experience that he wrote his Masters thesis on the subject, and dedicated himself to helping women who've suffered OASIs. Women all over the world lose their jobs, marriages, sex lives and dignity as a result of these injuries. And GPs, health visitors and midwives, who are often the frontline responders, are not always equipped to help, due to inadequate training and resources. Recognising this, MASIC has started a number of support groups across the country for women to meet others with similar problems, share coping strategies, and enjoy each other's company without fear of misunderstanding or stigma. MASIC also campaigns for better information around childbirth; women should be warned of the risks of anal sphincter injuries, Mike believes, as well as given information on how to prevent them. Part of his campaign is for every woman to have an appointment with a midwife at around 36 weeks pregnant where she learns about the risks of childbirth, including anal sphincter injuries. He also wants every woman to be offered a rectal exam (a finger in the bottom to check for damage) after a vaginal birth, to stop them going undetected. Mike has a knack for making people feel comfortable discussing these issues – he favours the word bottom instead of anus and poo instead of faeces. It's from Mike that I learn that we can all, whoever we are, help to break down this taboo of 'bottom problems', as he calls them, by finding words that we're comfortable with; we can dismantle the stigma and taboo by helping our friends, relatives and, one day, daughters to be more open about these things so that fewer women suffer in shame and silence.

Treatment

Part of the problem in the UK is that treatment pathways for bowel problems like wind and faecal incontinence are chaotic. If you have any symptoms, it's recommended that you see a specialist gynaecologist or pelvic health physio as soon as possible. NICE also recommends that women with third- or fourth-degree tears should have access to psychological support if they want it; these injuries can take a long time to heal, psychologically speaking, and talking to a professional can make a huge difference.

If you see your GP or midwife about your symptoms, prepare for the fact that they may not know much about anal sphincter injuries or faecal incontinence; be persistent in getting help, and listen to your instincts. GPs and midwives really do want to know if there's anything wrong with your bowel, so they can help you before things get worse. If the idea of a rectal exam horrifies you, remember it's just another routine procedure for the person who's doing it.

Sally's first birth ended with an episiotomy and a tear. As a keen sportswoman, she expected to get back to training quickly, but couldn't do high-impact exercise without needing a poo. Four months after the birth, a consultant diagnosed a third-degree tear:
'I'd assumed that, because I had strong abs, I had a strong pelvic floor – but it seems that strong abs can almost

compensate for a weak pelvic floor. I was raring to go after the birth and signed up for a mums and bumps fitness group. At an appointment beforehand they asked about my bladder, but I had no problems with my bladder at all. And, as long as I'd done a poo that day, and as long as I wasn't doing any impact stuff, I was OK. But I was doing loads of abs work by the end of it. It was only then that I started running and had problems. I had this urgent need to poo and I couldn't do yoga without letting out a fanny fart.

'*I booked an appointment with a female GP and she couldn't find any sort of fistula (which could have explained the fanny farts), but said I had a really short space between my vagina and my rectum now, and that loads of scar tissue had pulled it together. The walls, she said, felt incredibly thin between the two. I knew that fanny farting was unusual for me, so I was ready to offer it up to my GP, but I think a lot of women would rather put up with it out of embarrassment.*

'*My doctor referred me to a consultant, and I had an intensive course of physio. The NHS physio said I shouldn't have been doing any of the abs stuff and shouldn't have been running. A mistake people make is to focus on the bladder but not on the bowel. Because my baby was back-to-back, all the damage was done to the posterior wall of the vagina and the external sphincter; they can now see the scar tissue. And there wasn't necessarily a fistula but it was so weak down there that I was trapping loads of air. I'm prone to tearing now, so I've been told that if I got pregnant again I would have a C-section.*'

Coping with symptoms

Women with bowel control problems tend to develop specific coping mechanisms to allow them to get on with their lives without too much disruption. MASIC provides the following advice for women learning to cope.

Toilet access – Disabled toilets are available to women with bowel-control problems; if you have any symptoms and worry about finding a loo in time, you can get a RADAR key from your local council or doctor, or you can buy them for a small amount from www.radarkey.org. A number of websites publish the details of all public loos online (see Resources), and a number of companies publish 'Just Can't Wait' cards, which you can use if you want to request access to a non-public loo, or are faced with a long queue.

Hygiene – It's ideal to wash the area with water in a bidet or a shower but this isn't always possible. You can get moist tissues or 'washlets' – like baby wipes but made from paper, so flushable – from most supermarkets to make hygiene easier. If you're at home, you can use a sitz bath to clean and soothe the area, or get a plumber to attach a hose sprayer to your loo's water supply – it's cheaper than loo roll, and better for you and the environment.

Loperamide – The drug everyone takes on foreign holidays (as the brand Imodium), loperamide slows down the passage of poo and makes for a thicker, firmer final product, which is easier to control. It's very safe – it can be taken long term for diarrhoea/loose stools if there is definitely no serious and undiagnosed underlying cause – but it might take a while to figure out the right dosage. Some women take it daily, others just when they need it. It comes in syrup or tablet form; the syrup is prescription only and best if you want small doses and to prevent constipation, while you can buy the tablets over the counter.

Diet – Adjusting your diet if you have any bowel problems can take time. Some women who struggle to control their wind find the low-FODMAP diet, which eliminates certain carbohydrates, to be helpful (see Resources). Others find high-fibre foods, beans, pulses and cabbage, and certain fruit like rhubarb, figs, prunes and plums problematic. The MASIC website lists other foods that may make symptoms worse, and it includes alcohol, caffeine, lactose, artificial sweeteners and spices. Foods contain both soluble and insoluble fibre; increasing the amount of soluble fibre and reducing insoluble fibre may help. For example, dried apricots, beans, chickpeas and peas all contain soluble fibre, while wholegrain cereals and wheat flour contain insoluble fibre.

Supplements – Natural supplements including peppermint oil, charcoal tablets, mint tea, cardamom seeds, aloe vera, acidophilus or probiotic tablets or drinks like Activia, kombucha or kafir may help to reduce wind, as could an indigestion medicine like Rennie or Pepto-Bismol.

Pelvic floor muscle training – Strengthening the sphincter muscles is essential to prevent leakage; see page 227, Pelvic Floor Strength Training.

Bowel training – Just as with urinary incontinence, it's possible to train your bowel to wait until you're ready to go. You need to progressively increase the time between getting the urge to go and emptying your bowel. If you do this alongside your pelvic floor muscle training, you should gradually reduce the urgency and improve your control.

Doing exercise – It's good to walk or do some form of exercise regularly, although things like running and heavy lifting might make leakage worse. The pelvic floor muscles are generally stronger in the morning, so if you can't avoid – or don't want to avoid – strenuous activity, it may be better to do it then. You can wear pads or buy supportive shorts in a quick-drying material, and always make sure you empty your bowel before you start.

Bowel emptying – If you do want to do something strenuous or just be sure you're not going to have an accident, a glycerine suppository, which you insert and leave in to bring on a bowel movement, is very good at emptying the lower bowel completely. Combined with loperamide, this can ensure you're symptom-free. Similarly, you can use micro-enemas or rectal irrigation to empty the lower bowel. These are things that a specialist continence nurse should advise you on.

Inserts – Like tampons for the back passage, a variety of disposable products are available to prevent leakage and provide reassurance.

Pelvic pain

It used to be that pelvic health physios saw more cases of weak pelvic floors than anything else. Now, I'm told, they see just as many if not more cases involving tight, painful, overactive pelvic floors which often manifest as pelvic pain.

This could be because women are more stressed and anxious today than in previous decades, or just because there is more awareness of the issue and the fact that it can be treated. Physiotherapists observe that pelvic pain – for example, during sex or when you wee – usually affects competitive, ambitious, anxious high-achievers. The condition is becoming more common in young women who have not yet had children; often, it's misdiagnosed as a urinary tract infection.

There are lots of reasons why pain around your vagina and pelvic area might persist beyond six to twelve weeks postpartum, including: overactive, tender or hypervigilant pelvic floor muscles, which respond too intensely as if to protect you; scarring of the perineum or scar tissue associated with a C-section; tense muscles that need releasing; nerve damage; and bone problems. Chronic pelvic pain happens after the original infection or insult – it's more like a memory of a traumatic event. And it can be a bit like the Princess and the Pea – a tiny sensation in the pelvis is given undue attention by the brain until it causes disproportionate levels of discomfort. The area of your brain that is responsible for receiving messages from your pelvic floor is tiny compared to most body parts, which is why signals are so often confused – the communications infrastructure simply doesn't allow for much nuance. To treat pelvic pain, you have to teach the brain not to over-react, a process known as down-regulation. There are things you can do for this yourself, for example massage (see page 207). If the pain does not go away, a pelvic health physiotherapist is the place to start (see page 180).

Overactive pelvic floor muscles
We are typically told to tighten and hold our pelvic floor

muscles to improve their function. If you have overactive (or hypertonic) pelvic floor muscles, the opposite is true; you need to learn to relax, not tighten, them. A good test is to see whether you can feel your pelvic floor lifting up and dropping down as you tense and relax the muscles. If you can't feel it dropping, your muscles may be over-tense and causing discomfort. Possible causes include physical and mental trauma as a result of pregnancy and birth, stress, instability elsewhere in the body that's making you grip with your pelvic floor, or bladder and bowel problems for which your pelvic floor is compensating. As with pelvic pain, it's possible to down-train the muscles so that they start functioning normally.

Pudendal nerve pain

Pain or numbness in the pelvic area can occur as a result of your pudendal nerve, the main nerve that serves the pelvis, getting squashed, damaged or irritated during birth. Symptoms include pain, numbness, hypersensitivity or pins and needles in your clitoris, labia, vagina, urethra, perineum or rectum, finding it difficult to sit down, and having problems with sex or going to the loo. Usually, any damage from the birth will resolve itself within a few weeks. It doesn't always, however, and it can even come back months or years after the birth. The pain responds well to physiotherapy and a women's health physio should be trained to identify and treat it.

Painful or difficult sex (dyspareunia)

Dyspareunia, the technical term for difficult or painful sex, affects around 40 per cent of women in the six months after they give birth (and a whopping three-quarters of sexually active women at some point). Despite this, it is perpetually misdiagnosed, mismanaged, trivialised, neglected and ignored, according to Kate Walsh, at Liverpool Women's Hospital.

The causes can be physical and emotional, but it's often a combination of the two, with a complicated interplay between them – which can make the symptoms challenging to manage.

Even though you experience the pain in your pelvic area, Kate explains that the pain is generated by your brain, which can overreact, telling all of your muscles to tighten up and be on red alert (see page 179). Physical causes include a vaginal tear or perineum that hasn't healed properly, an infection, cystitis or haemorrhoids. The brain interprets these as threats, the muscles and soft tissues react to guard against them, and then they start to anticipate threat, becoming hypervigilant. This intensifies the problem and creates a cycle that can be difficult to break. Some women can also experience an involuntary muscle spasm (known as vaginismus) that makes penetrative sex difficult. Emotional causes include relationship issues, work and financial stress, depression and anxiety.

Episiotomies seem to contribute to painful sex more than spontaneous tears, but it's not clear whether their impact is any worse in the long run. Another possible cause of pain is breastfeeding, or progestogen-only pills, which can cause dryness that makes sex more painful; experts wish the NHS gave all new mums a tube of lube in their welcome pack. Until they do, buy yourself some.

If the problem persists, see your doctor for a referral – or refer yourself – to a pelvic health physiotherapist (and, if necessary, a psychotherapist), who can treat the pain by exploring its origins. A physiotherapist will ask questions about your bladder and bowel function as well, which may not be something you'd expect to be relevant, but it is all part of the complex jigsaw. Alternatively, you can also try massaging yourself at home (see page 207).

Kate Walsh, pelvic health physiotherapist, on treating pelvic pain:
'When I assess, we explore the pain and, crucially, the body's response to the pain. We look into whether it is physical or emotional in origin – with a significant overlap of both. We identify the onset of the pain and potential triggers. It is also important to assess bladder and bowel function, which is often key and not something that many women put in the same compartment as the pain they're experiencing. I look at posture and how they move. Exploring their breathing is also important, and then I'll do an assessment of the vulva and vagina, including the pelvic floor muscles. First, I explain to them what I'll be looking at when I examine them – including the ligaments, muscles and tendons, the support offered by the fascia, and how everything connects. Some people have said to me, "Oh! And there was me thinking it was just a hole." If you start sweeping around and feeling for tension or gaps, shortened muscles, lengthened muscles, the range of movement, and then turn it into something they can see and understand, that goes a long way to helping their recovery – whether it is releasing, training or desensitising. I often remark on how I could potentially forage around for half an hour within a pelvis, assessing, understanding and deciding on treatment; it isn't just a quick in and out to assess the pelvic floor muscles! Having said that, it should not be uncomfortable for the patient, and prior education on*

*the reasoning behind the examination helps people under-
stand and feel in control of the assessment [...] It's also
about the external genital area and vulva, looking at skin
condition, areas of sensitivity, tension and scarring. We also
assess the larger groups of muscles which help to stabilize
the pelvis externally, the piriformis, glutei, hamstrings, hip
flexors, inner thigh muscles and deep abdominals. We want
to realign people; rehabilitate balance and symmetry within
muscles working across joints to re-train normal movement. This, in turn, can provide benefit to down-training
and desensitising the perineal area that is so often on red
alert. I teach women to do their own perineal massage, in
conjunction with diaphragmatic breathing, familiarising
themselves with their own body in an attempt to remove the
fear and help release the pelvic floor muscles and normal-
ize the sensitivity. A lady yesterday said to me, "So you're
saying my muscles are too tense to tense?" "That's exactly
what I'm saying," I said.'*

How to relax

When we get stressed, our bodies generate muscle tension
– it's our way of getting ready to flee, or fight. Other emotions, like fear, grief, anxiety and anger can trigger the same
response. Physical activity helps to drain that tension, but
if we can't get out for regular exercise, what else can we do?
Laura Mitchell was an antenatal teacher and physiotherapist
in post-war Britain who, back in the 1970s, identified the
importance of relaxation for both mind and body. She started
offering lunchtime 'relaxation' classes in Lambeth, for 'over-
tired city workers', as well as a correspondence course, and
the relaxation technique she pioneered is still in use today.

Known as the Laura Mitchell Relaxation Technique, or the Mitchell Method, it involves methodically repositioning parts of your body so that you end up in a more relaxed posture, relieving the muscle tensions produced by stress. The UK's professional network of Pelvic, Obstetric and Gynaecological Physiotherapists, the POGP, recommends it for anyone with a painful bladder, interstitial cystitis, anal pain, vaginismus, painful intercourse or other problems relating to a high-tone pelvic floor – although it can be useful for anyone, from women in labour to drivers on long journeys. (See Resources for a link to a download published by the POGP that outlines how to do it.)

Methods for pain relief

Gentle massage and relaxation techniques can help to relieve the pain of muscle spasms and re-educate your body so that it no longer senses pain or danger where, in fact, there is none.

Perineal massage

Physiotherapists recommend perineal massage before sex for women who experience pain on penetration or orgasm.

> Lie back with your knees bent and feet flat. Use a small amount of lubricant and gently apply pressure to the perineal body, between the back passage and the opening of the vagina, for 30 to 90 seconds; this helps loosen the tissue and increase blood flow.

Internal massage

Physiotherapists recommend starting with external massage then progressing internally to relax and lengthen the muscles of the pelvic floor if they are tight. Internal massage can also be used to identify sore spots and release them by applying firm but gentle pressure to the muscle.

> Lie back with your knees bent, feet flat. First work externally. Use some lube and move in circular strokes around the vulva and inner and outer labia. Then apply sustained pressure to the perineal body, starting with as little as five to ten seconds. Next, imagine the area around your vagina as a clock; your pubic bone at 12 o'clock, and anus at 6 o'clock. Insert your finger to a depth of about an inch and start at 6 o'clock. Move gently and slowly anticlockwise to 1 o'clock, probing for sore points as you go. Then go the other way, clockwise, from 6 o'clock to 11 o'clock. When you hit a sore point, apply pressure – very gently, as these muscles and tissues are highly sensitive – for between 30 and 90 seconds. Then move on. You can go as far as four inches into the vaginal canal to assess the different muscles of the pelvic floor, but be careful to be gentle with yourself. You never want to probe the area between 11 and 1 o'clock, because the urethra and bladder are there.

Sex toys for pain relief?

They may appear to come from opposite ends of the pleasure spectrum, but sex toys and pelvic floor therapy can share the stage when it comes to releasing painful muscles and even softening scar tissue. If you find sex painful because your muscles are too tense, or you have particular spots that are tender, dig out your vibrator – or invest in a little bullet vibrator or a dedicated pelvic wand.

There isn't yet much evidence for sex toys specifically in relation to pelvic pain, but vibration is used widely by therapists including chiropractors and physios elsewhere in the body to loosen tight muscles – so why not in the vagina and perineum as well? A number of pelvic health physiotherapists suggest their clients take bullet vibrators home to desensitise and down-train the sore spots – and one American physio even designed a vibrator specifically for this purpose.

Dr Amanda Olson was working as a paediatric neurologist when she fell 12 metres on a camping trip, dislocating her coccyx and damaging her pelvic floor's muscles, ligaments and tendons. A pelvic health physiotherapist oversaw her complete rehabilitation – but the accident left her with a passion for treating pelvic health, so she retrained as a physiotherapist. She has since developed a number of products, made by the American women's health retailer Intimate Rose, which are designed to help women relieve pelvic pain at home – including vibrating and non-vibrating versions of the pelvic wand, a small, curved silicone snake that's designed to reach the superficial and deep pelvic floor muscles. You gently sweep around with the wand until you find a sore spot (or 'trigger point'). You then gently press the sore spot using the wand 'with the same firmness you would use to check a tomato for ripeness', as the Intimate Rose website says. You can try using the same principle with a small vibrator.

Pelvic physiotherapists also use dilators – which look no different to a sex toy – to help women who have tense or overactive pelvic floor muscles to relax them; dilators don't stretch the vagina but train the muscles to relax while you're inserting something. The technique isn't just for new mums – a lot of young women, those experiencing changes around the menopause, or athletes with hypertonic pelvic floors find their muscles benefit from what experts call a vaginal trainer or dilator.

Prolapse

The change brought about in me by childbirth can be summarised as follows. Before, I didn't know what a prolapse was; now, I know that half – half! – of all women are likely to have one at some point in their lives, and I want to relay this fact to as many women as possible, so they can take action to minimise their risk.

The taboo that surrounds this common condition is unhelpful and misleading; the pelvic organs naturally drop down a bit in all of us as we age, and some people experience this worse than others. There isn't even a precise academic definition for what constitutes a pelvic organ prolapse; 'normal' pelvic organ support varies with age and the number of children you've had. Some women will never have problems, some will have no symptoms for years, while others will have symptoms that appear straight after birth. Since 2019, NICE has recommended physiotherapy as the first line of defence, and for good reason; it works.

Women often describe a prolapse as having a tampon that's fallen down, or heaviness in the vagina. The pelvic floor muscles and ligaments become stretched and weakened to the point that they're not able to keep your pelvic organs – bladder, uterus and bowel – in the correct place. As a result, one of these organs, often the bladder, bulges down, either into your vagina (in the case of the bladder and uterus) or your anus (in the case of your rectum). While this sounds dramatic, many prolapses are mild, and manageable with physiotherapy alone.

It was a conversation about a prolapse that inspired this book, in fact, and helped me overcome my own pre-programmed sense of taboo. My friend Ella is a fit and strong, clear-eyed and pink-cheeked mother of two energetic boys; hers is the sort of fresh beauty you only get from a love affair with the outdoors. If she isn't mountain biking, she's running in the hills or kayaking. In short, she is not an obvious candidate for a prolapse. But in the year I got to know her, shortly after my own son's birth, she was struggling with a cystocele, a prolapsed bladder, that her GP refused to take seriously even though she kept going back. Eventually, she resorted to a private appointment with a pelvic health physiotherapist. The physio told her what she needed to do, she applied herself to the exercises as prescribed and, within a year, was back to full strength.

If we can break the taboo surrounding prolapses now, we will start to break down the system of neglect that denies women preventative care and leaves their symptoms to worsen with age until they reach breaking point. With our ageing populations and growing waistlines, scientists predict an epidemic of pelvic floor disorders, and urge younger women to invest time and energy now to prevent problems in the future.

Ella spent six months going back and forth to her GP with symptoms of a prolapsed bladder before taking matters into her own hands; she now runs 10 kilometres without any issues:
'I remember wearing the baby in a carrier to my six-week

appointment with the GP and saying something doesn't feel right down below – it feels like I've got something coming down. The doctor didn't examine me. She just said it's very early days, come back in three months. I went back at five months, again with the baby in the carrier. This time she did have a quick look and said she didn't see anything, but to come back again in a couple of months. Sometime after that appointment, I worked out that it felt worst on the days when I was carrying the baby furthest, so I started putting him in a pram. The next time I went back to the doctor, she finally gave me an information sheet about prolapses. It said, if you think you've got a prolapse, avoid carrying your child. Three times she'd seen me wearing my baby and failed to mention the documented recommendation that I stop doing so.

'It really did affect my quality of life and the way I was able to think about myself as an active person. It's faded now but I was really cross at the time, that I had presented with a very definite problem and kept being sent away. I feel that more proactive support from an earlier stage could lead to much more successful outcomes that don't require such dramatic interventions down the line. In other countries, that care is provided as standard, and I think it would give mothers here a much stronger start.

'The GP immediately started talking about how it could be fixed by medical intervention. There was a lot of controversy about vaginal mesh in the media, and I said there was no way I was going to consider it unless I'd gone through all other options. I did some research online and found that you need a specialist physiotherapist. I found one nearby and, even though it was £80 for an hour, I decided to pay that money – and it was amazing. She went through my whole history, and did a more in-depth exam than the doctor, who

just had a quick look. She got me to practise pelvic floor exercises, to make sure I was able to isolate the right muscles, helped me to tweak the way I was doing things, then gave me a set of exercises that were tailored to me. The important part was that I was able to actively release the muscles, rather than letting them fade out. She also said that I need to be doing the pelvic floor exercises while I'm doing other things, like going up and down the stairs. With that guidance, and with my decision to not carry the baby so much, I became a lot more stable.'

Prolapse symptoms

Symptoms go beyond feeling heavy around the vagina and as if something is dragging or coming down below. They can include backache, feeling sore in your lower abdomen, problems with urinary incontinence, bowel problems including constipation, getting frequent urinary tract infections, and pain, leaking or discomfort during sex. To get a diagnosis through the NHS, you'll need to ask your GP to examine you. You can ask at your practice if there's a GP who specialises in women's health. You may also want them to examine you standing up, if that's when you have symptoms. They should then refer you on to a specialist, depending on the severity of your case. Alternatively, you can make a private appointment with a uro-gynaecologist, or a pelvic health physiotherapist (the more affordable option), who will be able to make a diagnosis.

Types of prolapse

Unless you've studied pelvic anatomy, understanding exactly

TYPES OF PELVIC ORGAN PROLAPSE

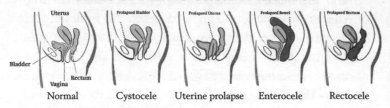

Normal   Cystocele   Uterine prolapse   Enterocele   Rectocele

what is going on down below if you have a prolapse is not always easy. These are the prolapses most commonly experienced by women at some point in their lives after giving birth.

Cystocele [pron. SIS-toe-seal] – The most common type of prolapse, when the bladder bulges into the front wall of the vagina.

Uterine prolapse – In this situation, the uterus bulges or hangs down into the vagina.

Enterocele [pron. EN-tur-oh-seal] – This occurs when the small intestine compresses the upper vagina.

Rectocele [pron. REC-toe-seal] – When the rectum, the final section of the large intestine just above the anus, prolapses, it usually manifests as a bulge in the back wall of the vagina (see page 189).

Treatment

Prolapses have been recorded for millennia. In Ancient Egypt, doctors would rub the patient's body with petroleum, manure and honey to fix it. Over a thousand years later, in around 400 BC, a contemporary of Hippocrates, the founder of Western medicine, liked to irrigate the prolapsed uterus with wine, or hang the woman by her feet and jiggle her upside down for three to five minutes so that gravity could do its work. Hippocrates himself believed that the risk factors for a prolapse included wet feet, over-exertion, fatigue, sexual excesses and – last but not least – having children. Incidentally, Hippocrates' son-in-law favoured inserting half a pomegranate into the vagina as a cure.

Medical approaches to fixing prolapses have, thankfully, advanced, although not as far as you might hope. In the UK, roughly 10 per cent of women will undergo surgery during their lifetime to strengthen the tissues around the prolapse with stitches, but often the operation only fixes it temporarily; around a third of women develop another prolapse within just a few years of surgery. Studies support conservative management – in particular physiotherapy and non-invasive treatments rather than surgery – because surgery fails, and is hard to fix again, whereas physiotherapy and pessaries work. NICE recommends a supervised programme of at least 16 weeks of pelvic floor muscle training. You can also try wearing a supportive ring called a pessary that sits at the top of the vagina to support the womb and/or walls of the vagina. You won't notice you're wearing it, and you can leave it in all the time – including during sex – to manage symptoms and hold things in the right place while you strengthen the muscles surrounding it. Women who want to keep working out or running during their recovery, for instance, may find a pessary helpful, and can learn to put it in themselves.

Daily management

Until you strengthen the muscles, it's important to minimise the pressure you exert on your pelvic floor. Avoid having to strain on the loo – change your diet or take a supplement if necessary. When you lift something heavy, lift with your back straight and contract your pelvic floor muscles first (see page 179). Try to use a pram rather than a baby carrier where possible, and avoid standing for long periods of time. Avoid high-impact sports until you get professional advice, and try to keep your weight within a normal range. If you want to have sex but it's painful, try using lubricant and different positions until you find what works; sex won't make your prolapse any worse.

Mesh controversy

One of the most controversial medical interventions of recent years is the implanting of plastic mesh to treat prolapse and incontinence, introduced in 1998. This ill-considered surgery left many women around the world unable to walk, have sex or work due to persistent pain and infection, and led to several class-action lawsuits against Johnson & Johnson, which marketed them. The pharmaceutical giant has now paid out hundreds of millions of pounds in compensation and fines for putting profit ahead of women's health, and mesh implants are now treated as a last resort.

> *Carrie tore badly during her second birth, a VBAC delivery, but doctors and midwives never warned her of the problems she might encounter further down the line:*
> *'When I had my second, I was really committed to a natural birth. The baby was huge, so I was induced, but because she*

was so big they had to use forceps and I ripped very, very badly. Afterwards, the midwives said nothing about what the implications might be; nobody had that conversation with me.

'*Over the next couple of years, I became very, very constipated. It was like the whole of my pelvic floor dropped and I couldn't go to the toilet; it was like it would bulge down and I literally couldn't poo. It was so embarrassing, I didn't go to the doctor; I couldn't talk to anyone about it. I thought I had bowel cancer. Eventually, after being so uncomfortable for such a long time, I went to see the local GP who specialised in women's health. She gave me constipation medicine, and said it was anxiety. At the same time, I started bleeding constantly, alongside these other symptoms. I suggested it was the menopause – and it turned out I was right – but she said I was too young; erratic bleeding was normal. This went on for nearly a year. I kept going back, and she kept sending me away with medicine for constipation. She made me feel I was making a fuss about nothing. It was just awful, I couldn't exercise, I was finding it difficult to even go for a walk.*

'*A lot of the symptoms were the same as for ovarian cancer, so I got a private scan done, which came back clear. The GP had referred me to a gynaecologist, but it was a 12-month waiting list for an appointment. It was my mum who said I needed to go private to find out what was going on – for the kids' sake, because it was making me so anxious. So I got a private appointment with a gynaecologist.*

'*The experience was not a pleasant one. On examining me, he said, "It's very flappy flappy down there, but you'd expect that having had two children." He found I had a prolapse – probably as a result of the episiotomy. Faeces was backing up, so it felt like I needed to go but couldn't. I was relieved to have a diagnosis, but felt humiliated by the whole thing. He did, however, refer me to an NHS physiotherapist, and she was amazing. She said that a large proportion of elderly women in nursing homes are in those homes because they're incontinent, and they're incontinent because they didn't get the treatment for their pelvic floor that they needed when it could have had an impact. By being aware of what they need to do, a lot of women could avoid admission to nursing homes in old age. She gave me exercises, and lifestyle advice, and has taken me from barely being able to go for a walk to the point that I don't think about it on a daily basis anymore.*

'I just wish somebody had explained that this was a potential implication of the birth, so that I didn't spend years worrying that I had ovarian or bowel cancer while it got progressively worse. I don't think I've ever felt so low; I felt old, unattractive, that nobody understood what I was going through, and embarrassed to communicate about it – which is why I do now communicate about it, because if one person hears my story and it helps them, then it's been worth it.'

Getting help

It's time British women had access to the same sort of physical therapy that French women get after giving birth – specialist, one-on-one physio, paid for by the state, that ensures a woman's pelvic floor is fully rehabilitated before she's discharged from the system. Until that becomes a reality, women experiencing problems should think about the positive impact they could have on our system simply by speaking up.

A hidden problem

After my GP told me she wouldn't recommend treating my pelvic floor until we'd completed our family, I answered with a meek, 'oh, right', and skulked off with my tail between my legs.

Later, however, I was puzzled. Do you wait to rehabilitate a runner's injury because it *might* get better on its own and then they *might* injure it again? Her advice failed to take account of so many things: that I shouldn't have to put up with discomfort for years, especially during my first child's formative years; that strengthening my body now will better prepare me for birth next time round; that birth is not like an Etch-A-Sketch that erases for good all of your hard work, because muscles have memory; and that giving me the tools to strengthen my body now will prevent me from burdening the healthcare system with more complex problems in the future. It seems archaic and woefully short-sighted to deny help to new mums with pelvic floor problems on the basis that they might have more children one day.

Now pregnant with my second, if I have symptoms that are affecting my life after six weeks postpartum this time around I intend to badger and moan until I get a course of physiotherapy, and I won't take no for an answer. If necessary, I will be the woman my GP dreads. And, if the waiting list is too long, I will save money elsewhere in our life and pay for it. Anecdotally, obstetrics and gynaecologists estimate that doctors see only one-third of women with incontinence in the UK; two-thirds of the iceberg are hidden. If we give up at the first hurdle the NHS throws in our way, we'll be helping to mask the problem and supporting the status quo.

The importance of talking

After my unhelpful appointment with the GP at six months, I started to ask whether we as mums are doing enough to prioritise our post-birth recovery; sadly, I concluded, most of us are probably not. I'd read widely about my health during pregnancy, and later about my baby and its development. But I never read anything about my own physical recovery – until I started anxiously googling problems as and when they arose. I found it difficult to share my postnatal complaints with anyone, including my GP, and down-played physical symptoms because of an ingrained sense of shame.

It's not just me, and it's certainly not my fault – it's a societal thing. And society hasn't yet accepted the extent of the problem. As a lawyer who once worked for the Equality Commission told me, 'Because women aren't communicating these things, there doesn't appear to be a need.' But the need is huge, she said. The team behind MUTU System, the postpartum exercise programme, recently surveyed working women about symptoms of incontinence; a staggering 37 per cent of the women they surveyed had wet themselves in the last month at work. How can we achieve workplace gender equality without talking about things like that? Incontinence is not inevitable, but we're not getting the right healthcare. And it's not like we have a choice in the matter – we are, after all, the only ones who can give birth.

The law has not yet caught up with these facts; women lose jobs and suffer indignity and shame as a result of the taboo and stigma around their issues. But it's in our power to speak up and ask for help, demand more funding for our health system, lobby for change, and bring our children up to be aware of the issues and to discuss them more openly so they can come to the surface and be accounted for.

Chantal Davies, a professor of law, believes it is imperative that we somehow level the playing field:

'When we're talking about the actual event of giving birth and the lead-up to birth, the law is pretty good in compensating for the disadvantages women might face in work. But we haven't really caught up on the physical impact childbirth has on women throughout the rest of their lives and particularly in the workplace. Beyond birth there are huge physical implications that will carry on for the rest of a woman's life. You hear women saying, they're my battle scars and I'm proud of them. That's lovely, but some of the long-lasting impact on our bodies is really quite restricting in terms of how we live our lives in our middle and later years. There is a big discussion which is starting to happen now around women going through the menopause, and what can be done to compensate for that in the workplace. I think the same needs to happen in relation to the long-lasting physical impact of childbirth. We have to recognise that, biologically, women are still the only people who can have children, so there has to be some recognition of this; it's not treating women more favourably, it's just levelling the playing field.'

Navigating the healthcare system

Given the prevalence of pelvic floor problems, getting help can be remarkably difficult – especially if you don't have the money or desire to pay for it privately. I interviewed one GP who has suffered intermittent leaking on jumping, coughing, or shortly before her period, for five years. I asked her why she hadn't seen someone about it.

'I know what I'd have had to go through to get anything done,' she said.

In most parts of the UK, doctors act as gatekeepers to specialists like gynaecologists and pelvic health physiotherapists, who are often overburdened and under-staffed. As the same GP explained to me, 'You can have old patients with prolapses literally hanging out and you can't even get them seen. There's a degree of prioritisation going on where some doctors are thinking, we can wait and see if it gets better. That sort of explains it, but it doesn't excuse it. It is not acceptable in a developed country, where we should be responsible for everyone, rather than having to firefight when it gets really bad. And treating these issues early would take greater pressure off the NHS in the long run.'

Clare Bourne, pelvic health physiotherapist, sets out the ideal scenario:
'Currently, most women only discover their pelvic floor when they get pregnant, but that needs to change. Having a healthy relationship with the vagina, vulva and the pelvic floor needs to start in schools. Currently, we say, "don't have sex, and this is how not to get pregnant". No. We need to say, this is the vagina and the vulva, and this is how to keep them healthy. It's also important to get children pooing better. When a toddler poos, they usually squat. But we put them on a loo, so they go from squatting to sitting on a toilet, which is not the best way to poo; potties need to be low or have foot rests because the child needs to lean forwards with feet raised, like adults, to help the pelvic floor muscles to relax, which allow the bowels to empty – this is something I'll teach my own children to do.
'As young women and men, we then need to learn that our pelvic floor helps with sexual pleasure; it's the key to better sex. This can be a helpful incentive to doing pelvic floor exercises. We see a lot of chaps with premature ejaculation

or pelvic pain – these can be young men who are massively into body building. They often have really tight pelvic floor muscles which they can't contract and relax properly as they lack flexibility.

'And then during pregnancy, we might invest and see personal trainers, but we don't often go to see a woman's health physio. I want pregnant women to come to me the minute they have symptoms, and not when they're 35 weeks pregnant, because early intervention is so helpful. Currently, the midwives, doctors and health visitors seeing the pregnant and postpartum women are not trained in pelvic floor muscle checks. As physios, we sometimes feel like we are hitting our heads against a brick wall to be heard and for our role to be understood and recognised, but times are changing and for the next generation it will hopefully be different.'

What you can do

If the thought of discussing your sex life or bladder problems with a stranger makes you cringe, take heart from the fact that you're not alone; I've still not entirely overcome my natural prudishness, even when talking to women's health professionals. Remember that whoever you approach for help – your GP, midwife, health visitor, gynaecologist or physio – not only will they have seen it all before, but they also chose their job because they enjoy helping women like you.

Your GP – GPs should not dismiss your problem as normal. Each practice will usually have a doctor who specialises in women's health; ask to see them, and ask for a 20-minute appointment if you'd like an internal examination as a ten-minute slot is not normally long enough. Know also that they might have to meet certain thresholds in order to refer you; for example, you may need to have had the condition for a certain number of months, have received a leaflet about pelvic floor exercises, or been doing the exercises for a certain period of time. Prepare for your appointment by informing yourself of the NICE guidelines; sometimes it's not that doctors don't want to help, but that they don't know what they should be recommending. For stress urinary incontinence, for example, NICE now says you should have a course of physiotherapy as the first-line treatment – with no caveat as to how many more children you plan to have!

Self-refer – Not all specialist NHS services need a referral from a GP, although this depends on where you live. You can self-refer for physiotherapy in parts of the UK; Squeezy, the app designed by physiotherapists in the NHS to help women do their pelvic floor exercises, now also has a directory of physiotherapists (see Resources). The directory specifies whether they work for the NHS and, if they do, whether you can self-refer.

Private healthcare – It is a travesty that, in parts of the country, timely and effective physiotherapy is reserved for those who can afford it; being wind- and watertight through your twenties, thirties and forties should not be a luxury. However, for those considering private healthcare, there are a few things to consider. Going private for one appointment does not mean you need to stay private; one private appointment with a consultant gynaecologist might be all you need to get a referral to an NHS physiotherapist, for example. And some women I spoke to found that one appointment with a specialist pelvic health physio was all they needed to set them on the right track to recovery; once they knew what they needed to do, they had the motivation to see it through without supervision.

Share your concerns – Whatever your problem, there will be other women experiencing the same or a similar thing, and often women you already know. All of the problems discussed in this book exist within my friendship group. By opening up about pelvic floor problems, in particular when you're talking to new mums, your health visitor, or friends and family, you may find some helpful solutions. It took me two and a half years to understand and address my bladder urgency, simply because it was never explained to me well; if we talk about these things more openly, we start to understand them better, and save other people from going through them as well.

Inform yourself – Research shows that pelvic floor muscle training works much better when it is supervised, but if you don't or can't seek outside help, there are a number of books about pelvic floor problems, including *The Pelvic Floor Bible* and *Heal Pelvic Pain*. The brilliant website myconfidentbladder.org tells you almost all you need to know about behavioural interventions to end bladder incontinence. And YouTube offers countless pelvic floor muscle training videos – although go cautiously as many are not evidence-based. One of the video hosts that I can recommend is Kari Bø, a Danish professor, personal trainer, and world-leading researcher into pelvic floor health (see page 183).

> **Kate Walsh, Physiotherapy Manager at Liverpool Women's Hospital:**
> 'Sometimes the internet can freak you out, and be more

harmful than helpful, but if you want to go online to find a professional near you, it's a really useful tool.'

Alex Heath, clinical hypnotherapist, on the power of the mind when it comes to healing:
'It sounds a bit kooky, but one of the things I do as a hypno-therapist is encourage people to think about their vagina in a way that's pro health and repair. When we've got a problem down there, it's very natural to feel like our body has let us down and to feel bad about it. That often means we have an unconscious conversation with it that's frustrated and focused on the fact that it's not working. This brings a lot of tension, upset and disconnect, and we can begin to think about parts of our body as the enemy. Although I'm not suggesting that sending positive vibes to your vagina is going to resolve every issue, I do think it is an important part of the mix. The mind–body connection means that, when you're doing your exercises, you can make them more effective if you imagine the tissues becoming stronger and stronger. You might like to think of them as a favourite colour, or imagine the muscle changing colour as it becomes stronger and harder. You might like to think about the tissues knitting together, repairing, building and strengthening. Really use the power of the mind and its ability to visualise, and to feel good about it. Especially when it comes to re-establishing a sexual relationship, it's important to feel good about our bodies and to say, "you know what, my body has been through this horrendous journey, but it's survived and it's come back, and it's stronger than ever." Psychologically, we can experience post-traumatic growth – and our bodies can too. They can be stronger and more resilient when they come back from these things.'

Pelvic floor strength training

In her popular Pelvicore Technique video on YouTube, Professor Kari Bø wears hot pink head to toe and sets off her brown hair with a spectacularly contrasting bleached fringe. She is the doyenne of pelvic floor fitness, but the woman on my screen is not of this era, and nor is her exercise video, which pulses with tacky library music; it provides a welcome break from the consciously stylish yoga and Pilates videos of today.

Kari got a PhD for her thesis on pelvic floor muscle training back in 1990, long before it was in vogue, and the programme she has developed since is – unlike the vague NHS-recommended exercises – proven to work.

The Kari Bø exercise video I did was designed for expectant mums, but there was no gentle squeezing involved. As I watched, Kari barked her commands with a quirky Norwegian lilt: 'Up, up, stay there, stay on top,' she shouted, after initiating each pelvic-floor contraction. At one point, she called on me to contract my muscles so hard that I felt 'shivering inside'. And then, just as I thought I'd nailed it, she added the 'intensive contractions', which involved holding a contraction at maximum strength then somehow adding in short, sharp pulses of extra contractions on top of the long hold. (Disclaimer: some physios caution that doing these 'intensive contractions' could irritate your muscles if you have any sort of pelvic pain – although, confusingly, there are instances where you have to work through the pain to resolve it. See page 201 for advice on relaxing a muscle if you think yours might be too tight or in spasm and, if in doubt, see a pelvic health physio for an assessment.)

The workout Kari presented was intense, and bore little resemblance to the casual squeezes I'd spent two years doing without results. Kari left such an impression on me that, even when she's not there, I now imagine her barking out from under her peroxide fringe – 'Up, up, up, HIGHER, you can do MORE!' – whenever I contract my pelvic floor. And, within a month or so of doing it every few days, I felt a noticeable difference in my contractions, which quickly become stronger and more responsive – even though I was three months pregnant, which should have been making them weaker.

What is pelvic floor muscle training?

The goal is to have a pelvic floor that is meaty, strong and functional – meaning it can contract quickly when needed (for example, when you sneeze), have endurance (for control of your bodily functions, for instance) and relax. Strictly speaking, one contraction of the pelvic floor muscles involves both the contraction and relaxation; it's a cycle of work and rest. This is why all pelvic floor strength training must involve appropriate relaxation in between contractions. If you've ever got stuck in an awkward position with your baby that doesn't allow your arm to relax, you'll know how dysfunctional your muscles become after a period of constant contraction. It's no different with your pelvic floor; it needs to return to its resting tone (although it will never be entirely relaxed – when you're sleeping, your pelvic floor muscles actually contract more as the night goes on, as your bladder fills up, putting more pressure on them). And then when you wake up and start your day, it needs to get back into what Elizabeth Braga, a physiotherapist at Liverpool Women's Hospital, calls the 'pumping mode', where it can respond to whatever demands you throw at it.

If you have a weak pelvic floor, experts recommend doing a mixture of contractions that improve your muscles' strength, functionality, response times and endurance. 'Once you achieve a certain level of strength, it's less about making the muscles stronger and more about improving the connection between them and the brain to enhance their performance,' Elizabeth explained. I like to think of the different muscles, fascia and connective tissues as an orchestra, because it's not about how loud any of the instruments are, but about their timing, ability to work in concert, and the quality of the notes.

You can train up your pelvic orchestra by increasing the number of sets, repetitions, or the frequency of exercises, but also by doing the contractions alongside other activities, and playing with different positions where gravity can either ease off or increase the challenge. Once your muscles are functioning well, if you want to take the strength to another level, many physios recommend that you start combining pelvic floor contractions with loading exercises such as squats – or even walking up the stairs. Some physios also believe that you can use impact sports like running – or whatever it is you want to do – to build your pelvic floor strength (see page 179), as you'll be working the muscle and improving its function as you go.

Pelvic health experts bemoan the fact that health systems around the world give out watered-down, ineffective advice – 'just squeeze!'– to all pregnant and postpartum women, rather than giving proper, targeted help to those who really need it. It takes regular, hard work to reform muscles; the more intensive the programme, the better the results.

According to Dr Andrew Siegel, a urologist who has authored numerous books on the subject, we are in the throes of a 'Kegel renaissance'. When the American gynaecologist Arnold Kegel first pioneered pelvic floor strength training in the early twentieth century, the exercise regimes he devised would have made even the most committed athlete pale, such was the focus and intensity they required. It is from him that Kegels – pelvic floor muscle contractions – take their name. Kegel's death in 1945 plunged the world back into a new dark age for the pelvic floor, which ended only recently, Siegel says. Today, we have new biofeedback devices and electrical trainers coming onto the market every year, a passionate tribe of pelvic health physiotherapists fighting Arnold Kegel's corner, and scientists pioneering research and pelvic modelling that will make childbirth safer for us all.

How to do pelvic floor muscle training

1. Isolate your pelvic floor muscles

The easiest way to find your pelvic floor muscles is to imagine you're stopping your wee mid-flow (while not actually doing so – you don't want to confuse your bladder), or holding in a fart. If you can't locate the muscles, breathing can help; take a deep breath in, then on the out-breath imagine you're drawing up a tampon inside yourself. Your buttocks should stay relaxed. Practise contracting the muscles on an out-breath until you're confident that you've isolated them.

2. Contract and release

As soon as you can feel the muscles, start doing exercises when you're upright; simply standing up makes the pelvic floor muscles work twice as hard than they do when you're lying down. Kari Bø recommends you stand with your feet hip-width apart, feet turned out, and put your hands on your bum. Squeeze your buttocks to check that they're soft and loose – and make sure you maintain that relaxation in your bum throughout the exercises. (If you can't, you're doing the exercises wrong and need to work on isolating the internal muscles again.) You then try to contract the muscles around the urethra, vagina and rectum; tighten, lift, hold it for a few seconds, and relax. Take a deep breath, exhale, then repeat. You can build the intensity of your contractions and the length of time you hold them for, and finish with bursts of short, sharp ones. For strength and endurance, experts suggest you aim for three sets a day, working up to 25 repetitions of five seconds of contraction and five seconds relaxation. The kicker – and why a lot of people give up – is that it can take up to three months for your symptoms to improve. Some physios object to the use of the word 'squeeze' for a pelvic floor contraction, because we associate it with other things; squeezing our buttocks, for example, or squeezing out a reluctant turd. Instead, try to imagine a contraction that starts around your back passage and comes forwards to tighten and lift around your vagina and, lastly, your urethra.

3. Targeted contractions

Physiotherapists recommend isolating the muscles in different places, so that you can tighten around the urethra, vagina and rectum independently. This might sound a bit far-fetched at first, but it's surprising how quickly you can get the hang of it. You can then imagine each is a lift shaft. Raise each area in stages up to the top floor, then lower it again. When you do your exercises, remember Kari Bø in her hot-pink gear guiding you through sets of both longer (five- to ten-second) holds, and shorter, sharper contractions; you should aim to do both – always at, or near to, maximum capacity – to increase both your strength and endurance.

4. Be mindful of functionality

Once you've got some strength back and you can contract and release the muscles while standing up, you should find that your muscles contract involuntarily when you walk or bear weight. If you do lift something heavy and you can feel the muscles struggling, get into the habit of contracting them before you bear the weight; by doing that, your toddler or laden car seat becomes part of your training regime. As physios say, unless your brain can coordinate these contractions while you're actually doing stuff, they're not helpful and, worse, you could end up injuring the pelvic floor structures. It's like people at the gym who are 'all show, no go', as Antony Lo says, who look buff but can't do anything much with it. Try to stop what you are doing before you have symptoms like leaking, but equally don't be afraid of putting your pelvic floor to the test, because you can improve it by using it. You may need to be more careful if you have a prolapse; a pelvic health physio will be able to guide you.

> *Antony Lo on pelvic floor training:*
> 'You can beef up your pelvic floor muscles, no problem with doing that, but the problem is the assumption that by having stronger muscles you're going to know how to coordinate them without thinking about it, for example, when you're running – and that can take practice. It's very reductionist to say that, to strengthen the pelvic floor, the squeezes are all you've got to do.'

Tools for strengthening your pelvic floor

If you want to buy a gadget, but haven't yet seen a pelvic health physio, consider spending the money on an assessment instead. If and when you then spend the money on a device, you'll at least know that you're using it correctly and doing the optimum exercises for your needs. If you do decide to go ahead and buy one, there is a huge variety available – and some even manage to make pelvic floor exercises fun.

'One of the best biofeedback tools is a penis.'
Kate Walsh, Liverpool Women's Hospital

Biofeedback tools (for example, Elvie) – A slick, pocket-sized trainer, the Elvie is one of the better-known tools on the market; it tells you what to do, gives you tips on doing exercises correctly, and monitors your progress. With its little tail, it looks oddly like a sperm cell – but other than that strange coincidence the design and materials are lovely and it is fun; when I use it, I feel like I'm back in the nineties playing Tetris, only with my vagina operating the controls. You pop the Bluetooth-enabled device inside you and connect it to your mobile phone via an app that tells you what to do. There is limited evidence to show that it makes a difference when compared with standard pelvic floor muscle training, but research has shown that it makes women do their exercises more often. If investing in something beautiful but also functional will help you adhere to a training programme, then a device like the Elvie could help; not sticking to a training programme is, after all, the most common reason for failure. Kate Walsh advises you treat a biofeedback tool as you would jumping on the scales each week at Weight Watchers – a helpful tool for motivation and monitoring your progress.

I have an Elvie Trainer – the company gave it to me to try – and I use it intermittently, as Kate suggests. Having used it to help establish that I was doing my pelvic floor exercises correctly, I liked the freedom of doing them anywhere. And, as I've become stronger, I've started to do them on the move – when walking, stretching, or even carrying my toddler. And then I return to the Elvie periodically, to see how I've improved.

Jade eggs – In Ancient China, the pelvic floor was revered as the source of a woman's primal energy force. Queens and concubines allegedly strengthened theirs by weightlifting with jade eggs, but kept the practice a secret, fearing what would happen if the power of the pelvic floor fell into the wrong hands. Gwyneth Paltrow is the most famous proponent of jade eggs today, selling them for £60 each on her website, goop. Their alleged properties include cleansing, improving orgasms, chi and vaginal tone, and rebalancing hormones. But some experts say using a jade egg is a bad idea. Firstly, jade is a porous rock, so it could harbour bacteria. Secondly, leaving the egg inside you for hours at a time, as goop once suggested in a controversial blog post, could teach the pelvic floor muscles to contract continuously, which isn't good for them; when you do pelvic floor muscle training, you should tense and then fully release. Lots of women do enjoy them, however, so if you really like the idea of using a jade egg, it's recommended that you see a physio first, who can tell you how to make it work for you.

Kegel weights – If you like the sound of vaginal weightlifting, you can also get medical-grade silicon or plastic products that doctors recommend. Kegel8, for example, makes vaginal cones, which are an affordable way to monitor your progress, and are available on prescription. There is no evidence to suggest that using weights in your vagina is more effective than just doing pelvic floor muscle training without them, but if putting one in for 15 minutes once or twice a day is easier than doing the exercises, then they could help you. You place a cone or ball just inside your vagina whilst standing and you use your pelvic floor muscles to bring it back up when you feel it slipping. Usually, you move onto a smaller or lighter cone as your muscles get stronger. Some people recommend using them in the shower initially, while you build up your strength. Used like that, weights like cones can help with endurance, but you need to rule out problems with an overactive pelvic floor first.

Electrical stimulators – In some European countries, it's routine practice for women to have their pelvic floor muscles stimulated by electrical pulses after childbirth. Bursts of small electrical current from a probe in the vagina cause the pelvic floor muscles to contract, which may be helpful if you can't contract your muscles at all. If you don't like the idea of a vaginal probe, you can also get stimulators that attach externally, or even a pair of toning shorts. There isn't much evidence to support them: a 2017 Cochrane Review found that electrical stimulation is 'probably' better than no treatment, but couldn't say whether it's as good as pelvic floor muscle training. And some experts worry that stimulation only moves the muscles, it doesn't strengthen them. In the UK, electrical stimulation is used selectively by physios and urogynaecologists. You can purchase electrical stimulation machines such as the Kegel8 Pelvic Toner online, but physios caution against this. 'I hate it when I see someone who's spent money they can't afford. There's so much misinformation. If you can do a voluntary contraction, you don't need to spend money,' one said. And a lot of women mistakenly think they can put the device in, sit back and relax while it strengthens.

It doesn't work like that, physios say; you need to do your exercises at the same time for it to work. NICE guidelines state that electrical stimulation should only be considered alongside pelvic floor muscle training if you can't actively contract your pelvic floor, and even then only to help with motivation. The French may swear by it, but until there is more conclusive scientific evidence, you're unlikely to find it widely recommended by professionals in the UK.

The French approach

Every French mother, including those who give birth by Caesarean section, is offered a course of individual physiotherapy sessions to reeducate her pelvic floor – *la rééducation du périnée* – and another set of physiotherapy sessions to rehabilitate her abs and core. As the French physiotherapist Eve Carré told me, 'People who have children can't ignore it.'

I boggled at a friend's descriptions of the one-on-one sessions she had with her physiotherapist in France. All of the exercises she learned were tailored to her needs. The physio had spotted that her urethra was sitting low, which was responsible for the pain during sex. To treat it, she taught my friend to do a complex exercise known as the *pelleteuse*, or digger, where she had to mimic the action of a digger with the muscles surrounding her urethra and vagina. Her progress, meanwhile, was monitored by an electronic probe. And by the end of the course, she had no pain anymore.

In general, pelvic floor rehab starts around six weeks postpartum in France, although some midwives encourage women to wait until they have stopped breastfeeding; your ligaments naturally become tighter as the hormone relaxin leaves your body. Once the rehabilitation is underway, Eve Carré explains that mothers across the Channel can expect to make a full recovery from postnatal incontinence within weeks. In a typical case, a French woman will attend ten sessions over six to eight weeks, in which time moderate incontinence will be resolved. Almost all women understand the importance of the pelvic floor, she said, and having individualised sessions with experts reduces the muscles' recovery time compared with self-guided recovery.

Bladder skill training

I was three months pregnant for the second time when John DeLancey pointed me to the interactive website that his colleague, Dr Janis Miller, had built, called myconfidentbladder. com. If you have any sort of urge incontinence, he said, just spending half an hour digesting the information on this site could dramatically improve your symptoms. I knew by this point that the bladder was a muscle, but even then his statement made no sense to me – what mysterious information could he be talking about? As soon as I got off the phone with him, I spent half an hour on this quirky little website, and it was transformational. The site draws on Janis Miller's 20 years of research and practice in the field of incontinence and pelvic health. It gives you skills that can prevent leaking when you cough or sneeze, allows you to find out if you're drinking too much, and teaches you to control your urge to wee if your bladder is not truly full. This website alone, which is cute and imaginative, was shown to reduce women's incontinence symptoms by 50 per cent in half of the women who used it – which makes it as effective as medication, so well worth thirty minutes of your life.

Within days of following Janis' recommendations, I didn't need the loo at night for the first time in over three years, and I was confident, even with a full bladder, that I could sneeze, cough or laugh without accident – even with the pregnancy hormones and a growing uterus inside me.

The traditional method of bladder training starts with a patient completing a three-day urine diary, measuring liquid in and liquid out, as a physiotherapist requested I do back when I was sleepless and struggling with a young baby. The physio was not wrong to suggest it, and there are various reasons why urine diaries are an important tool, but for me Janis' website would have sufficed – and has been a far easier (not to mention cheaper) way of solving my urgency problems.

What's normal?

Everyone is different but a normal bladder can hold 400 to 600 millilitres of urine, and on average people empty their bladders four to seven times a day, according to Guys' and St Thomas' NHS Trust, or roughly every three or four hours if you ask Janis Miller. A typical wee should contain around 250 millilitres of liquid – which equates to an average 20 seconds of flow. This is what you're aiming for – so when you next need the loo but find it's a tiny trickle, you'll know it was your brain and bladder tricking you.

Regaining bladder confidence

The best thing about bladder training is that a basic understanding of how the bladder works, and knowledge of simple techniques, can have a tremendous and instantaneous effect.

The knack – The knack is what professionals call the art of tensing your pelvic floor muscles just before you sneeze, cough, laugh or pick up a heavy child; it is one of the simplest and most effective things you can do for stress incontinence, in combination with pelvic floor muscle training. Before pregnancy, you probably didn't need to do this because your muscles had much better tone. Now, however, just like your abdomen, your pelvic floor has lost its tone and elasticity, so it needs extra help. By consciously providing extra tension, you can prevent leaking, and with practice, it becomes second nature. Experts suggest practising tensing the muscles and coughing when you have an empty bladder at first. As you get better at it and your muscles get stronger, you should be able to cough without leaking, even with a full bladder, and eventually it'll become a reflex.

Night wakings – A lot of women feel like their bladders wake them up during the night because they need a wee. What's more likely is that waking up triggers your urge to wee. After all, it's not as if you were about to wet the bed just before you woke up, so why the rush? The cause of this is often an over-excited bladder. Rather than obey it and go to the loo each time, even though your bladder isn't full, calm your bladder by sending a message to your brain; think of it like Morse code. Gently flex and relax your pelvic floor four or five times; doing so inhibits the urge to go. Continue this training when you wake up in the morning by not rushing straight to the loo. Tell your bladder to calm down, and go to the loo when you're ready. Your bladder should soon take note and stop being so demanding.

Daytime urges – If it feels like you constantly need a wee, or can't control it when the urge suddenly strikes, for example, when you put your key in the door, it's likely that you can learn to control these urges with a little practice. Janis suggests you think of your bladder as a hyperactive puppy; you need to calm it down. To do so, you first need to identify the triggers – what gets it excited? This might be putting your key in the door, leaving your desk, or entering the bathroom. You may find you have lots of different triggers. Once you've identified them, start doing four or five flicks of your pelvic floor muscles before (or, if it's too late, when) the urge strikes. This tells your brain that you don't need a wee, and stops your bladder being so needy. If you persist with this and gradually increase the time between wees, your problematic puppy should start to calm down – although it may take a few months to see real results.

Avoid the double void – If you've already looked into this subject, you may have seen people refer to 'double voiding' – when you take another wee, right after the first. Janis and other experts recommend you avoid this because it can make the bladder even more twitchy by training it to go little and often. Instead, after you've done a wee (and shifted about on the loo seat at the end a bit, if you like, to check your bladder is well emptied), do some more gentle pelvic floor squeezes to tell your brain that you're done.

Don't drink too *much* – It's common now to carry a water bottle everywhere and to see regular hydration as a good thing – which it is. But the notion that you must drink six to eight glasses of water a day is a myth, based on an unscientific recommendation from 1945 which actually went on to state that most of that water could come from food. Urologists and sports scientists recommend that you drink when you are thirsty, rather than go out of your way to drink a certain amount just because that's what you're supposed to do; it is a myth that to leave it until you're thirsty is to leave it too late. Everyone is different, of course, but drinking more than you need could be contributing to your symptoms. I interviewed one physiotherapist whose client was drinking the recommended two litres of water per day and wondering why she needed the loo so often. It turned out that she was drinking two litres of water on top of her intake of coffee, tea and wine, and her bladder was simply having to produce too much urine.

Avoid irritants – Certain drinks are shown to irritate the bladder and promote urge incontinence. The list of things to try eliminating includes artificial sweeteners, alcohol, tea and coffee (decaffeinated as well), and cranberry juice. It's also possible that acidic foods (like citrus fruits), dairy products, chocolate and spicy foods (amongst other things) are contributing to the problem. Try eliminating likely culprits for ten days to see if it helps.

16

Core Strength

Core *noun*
- The basic and most important part of something
- The muscles around your pelvis, hips and abdomen that you use in most body movements

    Source: *Cambridge English Dictionary*

It's no coincidence that the word 'core' confers the vital essence of someone or something. In humans, our core is essential for our everyday movements and functions – standing up, sitting down, turning to see something, walking, breathing, going to the loo – and, while our babies are busy strengthening theirs to do things like roll over and sit up, fitness experts say we need to be doing the same with ours. In Chapter 12, I wrote about reconnecting with your core. Now, it's time to strengthen it. But before you head to the gym, heed the words of experts, who say that it's important to first master the basic exercise in Chapter 15, which involves contracting the pelvic floor and deep abdominal muscles whilst breathing out. 'In doing this you are locking down the first stage of retraining, laying the foundations for further rehab and strengthening,' says Kate Walsh.

Posture

Whether the problem is your tummy, your sore back, your pelvic floor or your shoulders, physical therapists are fairly well united in urging women to start by thinking about their posture – how you hold yourself during everyday activities. If you can get this right, you may find the other issues go away. It's a complex – and highly individual – task to correct someone's posture, but Wendy Powell, the founder of MUTU System, has six golden rules for good alignment:

1. High heels are messing with your natural alignment and prevent your pelvic floor from functioning optimally; wear your heels less and wear minimal shoes without a raised heel as much as you can.
2. Keep your bum strong to keep your pelvic floor working well – don't tuck your tailbone under and do squats to build your glutes.
3. Straighten (but don't lock) your knees when standing – straight legs work better.
4. Stop sticking your chest out; you want your ribs to stack in line with your pelvis – imagine dropping your ribcage back and down (see page 244).
5. It's counterintuitive, but sucking in your tummy all the time makes your abs weaker, preventing them from working naturally; to get stronger, muscles need to release as well as contract, so let them relax and don't keep pulling your tummy in.
6. Practise, and walk every day, being mindful of the above.

GOOD ALIGNMENT

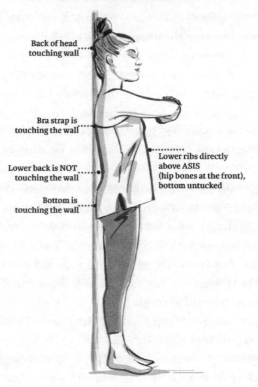

Back of head touching wall

Bra strap is touching the wall

Lower back is NOT touching the wall

Bottom is touching the wall

Lower ribs directly above ASIS (hip bones at the front), bottom untucked

Test for good alignment

Stand with your bum and back against a wall. Your spine should have a curve in it, so that your lower back is not touching the wall. Now consider where your bra strap is – is it touching the wall? If not, look at the position of your lower ribs at the front. Are they out ahead of the front of your hip bones? Bring your bra strap to touch the wall and notice how your ribs are now stacked above your pelvis. That's the alignment you want.

Back pain

> 'Has nobody noticed the embarrassing fact that science is about to clone a human being, but it still can't cure the pain of a bad back?'
>
> – Marni Jackson, author of
> *Pain: The Science and Culture of Why We Hurt*

One of the most common complaints of new mothers is back pain. The constant carrying, lifting and holding of a growing baby amounts to hard physical work, especially considering you've recently given birth. Over the course of nine months, your growing uterus gradually destabilised your body and changed your posture. You learned to move and hold yourself differently to accommodate your new shape and weight. Meanwhile, hormones loosened the ligaments and joints in your pelvis and spine. While the baby is now out and your uterus is the size of a large plum again, the other adaptations don't disappear overnight. You're also putting new pressure on your body by holding strange and uncomfortable positions when feeding or soothing your baby, lifting car seats and Moses baskets, humping prams up steps, and generally neglecting your own body in favour of your baby's. Six months into motherhood, I had the sort of biceps that inspire envy. The downside was that I felt twisted and unbalanced, tight and sore. You don't need to live with this feeling, and prevention is always better than cure.

Treatment and prevention

If you already have a sore back, the bad news is that modern medicine offers no panacea; in 2008, Australian researchers found that not one popular treatment has ever been shown to work well for lower back pain. Treating it effectively is more like a detective game that pieces together many different clues. In the absence of clear guidelines, the following advice is harvested from physiotherapists, chiropractors and osteopaths around the world.

Behavioural changes

Try early on to stamp out bad habits, such as always carrying your baby on one hip or picking it up without bending your knees. A lot of these things are fine when your baby weighs the same as a domestic cat, but less so when it becomes a 15-kilogramme sack of cat food, a transformation that happens remarkably quickly. If you get into good habits now, you will hopefully avoid problems and won't have to change ingrained behaviours further down the line.

Lifting – If you've ever lifted a car seat containing a child, you'll know they are designed for child – not parent – safety. When you can, squat down before you lift, engage your core – including abs and pelvic floor – breathe in, and lift by straightening your legs as you exhale. You may well engage your core muscles automatically, in which case don't overthink it. Try to carry things on both sides equally. And if your baby cries, don't always swoop down and pick them up; try squatting down in front of them and comforting them on the floor. When your baby becomes a toddler, encourage them to climb into their car seat or onto their chair; you can avoid a lot of lifting if you want to.

Cots – Repeatedly lifting a baby in and out of their cot can strain your back. Stand as near to the cot as possible, and keep the baby really close to you as you lift. Try to contract your core as you straighten up, and use your knees to lift, if at all possible. When your child gets bigger, you can get them to stand up before you lift them. And remember that if you engage your core correctly, that dodgy manoeuvre that was putting strain on your back and abs could become part of your strength training.

Maintain a normal BMI – Being overweight or obese means you're more likely to have back pain. If it's also the case that your muscles aren't strong because you're not exercising, your body is even more likely to struggle. If you are strong, however, your body is more likely to cope with any extra weight you're carrying around. Try to improve your diet (see Chapter 19) – eat plenty of healthy fats and protein but cut out sugars and reduce carbs, experts recommend walking regularly, and see the exercises below.

Warm baths

As the poet Sylvia Plath said, 'I am sure there are things that can't be cured by a good bath, but I can't think of one.' You can do stretches in the bath, or even put a tennis ball under your lower back or buttocks. Get the ball underneath any tight spots and, by lying on it, use gentle pressure to release them. There is no evidence to suggest that adding things like Epsom salts to your baths helps with pain – it's the warmth that's thought to be important (and if you had stitches, don't use Epsom salts until they've dissolved).

Feeding posture – However you feed your baby, try to sit upright as you do so, and don't hunch over; use cushions if necessary, or lie down rather than slouch in an awkward position.

Nappy changing – Get the nappy changing mat up at the right height so you're not stooping to use it; you should be able to stand up straight to change the baby.

Sleep positioning – If you sleep on your side, try putting a cushion between your knees; this aligns your hips and helps to keep your spine straight while you sleep, and may help with back pain during the day as well as at night.

Painkillers – Evidence suggests that paracetamol has little impact on back pain, so take ibuprofen, which is safe to use while breastfeeding.

Exercise for back pain

Doing just a few simple things like stretching and taking a decent walk each day can have a big impact on how your body and your back are feeling.

Walking – Walking has long been prescribed for back pain, and it also helps to keep you supple, strong and maintain a healthy weight. Research supports a 30- to 60-minute walk every few days, but it may not work so well if you are carrying a heavy baby on your chest that's pulling you off-centre. If you are carrying the baby, get a good sling, have it as high up on your body as possible, and move the baby onto your back as soon as advised (usually at around six months).

Yoga and Pilates – Yoga and Pilates are great for back pain, strengthening the muscles that support your spine and stretching out any tight ones. You don't even need to leave the house to do some yoga or Pilates for your back pain. Devise a short routine of poses and stretches to relieve some of the tension. It doesn't have to be too ambitious to start with – something you can do while the baby is nodding off, or before you get into bed each night. The NHS provides a free postnatal yoga video on its website, and also Pilates for back pain. You should know which postures feel good by doing them, but don't assume you can do whatever you did before, and make sure you avoid anything that overwhelms your abdominal muscles and causes your stomach to dome (see page 252).

Strength training – Whichever exercises you choose to do to strengthen your core, including the muscles that support your back, focus on maintaining balance and stability; if you don't feel strong enough to stay balanced and stable doing an exercise, modify it, or do something else until you get stronger and can return to it. To strengthen the deep abdominals that support your spine, draw your tummy button in towards your spine as you breathe out, and hold it for up to ten seconds. You can also strengthen your lower tummy by lying on your back with your knees bent and feet flat on the floor; breathe in and, on the exhale, raise one knee to your chest while drawing your tummy button towards your spine, then return the leg to the floor and do the other one. Repeat five to ten times.

Movement – Try pelvic tilts, when you lie on your back and tilt your pelvis back and forwards, flattening and arching the lower back. Or go on all fours and try what yogis call the cow cat pose: inhale and slowly arch your back, dropping your tummy towards the floor; hold this for a few seconds, then exhale as you round out your back as much as you can, dropping your head down and pulling your tummy in towards the sky.

The Body Mechanic's five-minute prescription for lower back pain

Sarah Keates Andrews is a biomechanics specialist who recommends the following three exercises for lower back pain. She cautions that if something doesn't feel right, you shouldn't do it; mobilising restricted tissue can be uncomfortable but should not be unbearable, so use common sense.

1. **Wall glides to mobilise the deep core muscle, the Quadratus Lumborum, that can cause tightness and pain in the lower back, hip and buttocks.**
(NB This is my absolute favourite for a stiff lower back; I tend to do it in the shower or while brushing my teeth.) Stand sideways-on to a wall with your feet a foot or two away from it. Now lean your shoulder against the wall. With your shoulders down and elbows at your sides, slowly let your hip drop towards the wall until you feel a restriction (not everyone does). Return to the start. You don't need to force the movement or hold the stretch, but nudge it gently. Repeat this ten times, ideally two to four times a day.

2. **Lying leg press to relax, lengthen and strengthen the gluteal muscles.**
Lie on your back and lift one knee up towards your chest. Put both hands behind the lower thigh then press your thigh

Wall glide   Lying leg press

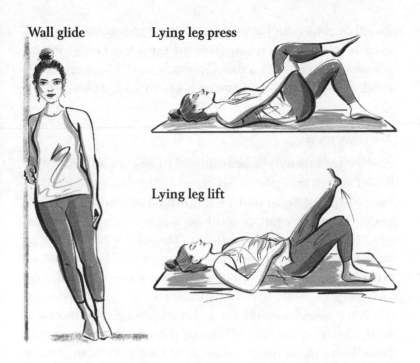

Lying leg lift

down into your hands, as if you were trying to straighten your leg out. Press at a comfortable resistance (around 20 per cent to start with); your leg should not move and your head and shoulders should be relaxed. Hold for 20 seconds, then release and repeat four times on each leg. Do this two to four times a day – in bed, if you like.

3. Lying leg lifts to activate hip flexors.
Lie on your back with one leg bent and the foot flat on the floor. Raise the straight leg and keep the toes pointing to the ceiling until the leg is in line with the opposite thigh, bracing your core as you lift. Raise for a count of two and lower for a count of two, and do enough reps to feel tired but

not exhausted. Aim for two sets of 15 to 20 repetitions comfortably (although you may start with just five or six) and do this two to four times a day. (You may need to place a hand under your lower back to ensure it's not lifting at all.)

Diastasis recti

Imagine your rectus abdominis, or 'six-pack', muscles as a pair of taut braces that previously ran straight down the front of your body, but separated to accommodate the baby. After pregnancy, these muscles come back together again, but the gap often doesn't close completely. The stretched connective tissue in between the muscles, known as the *linea alba*, can struggle to regain its elasticity and the tight corset that should encircle your abdomen remains weak and unsupportive. When the muscles and tissue are overwhelmed, the stomach can dome like a ridge line. This is commonly known as diastasis recti (diastasis meaning separation) and it has a lot of us in a stew. While mild diastasis can be asymptomatic, it can give us a less-than-flat belly, is linked to pelvic floor dysfunction and can lead to a muscular imbalance and chronic back pain.

Putting diastasis recti in context

The occasional doming that I noticed in my belly didn't bother me, until I started reading about it. 'The Postpartum Body Problem No One Talks About', read a headline in *Parents* magazine, which proposes exercise programmes, physiotherapy and, as a last resort, surgery. 'The serious injury no one is talking about', posited a blogger. I was told that this apparently taboo and problematic condition is responsible the world over for women still looking a bit pregnant long

ABDOMINAL MUSCLES

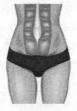 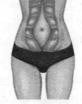

Normal   Diastasis Recti

after they've had their babies. Another website, Healthline, even led me to believe (mistakenly) that it could cause a hernia.

I leaped onto the floor to perform the test for diastasis recti, doing half a sit-up and feeling to see whether I had a gap of more than two centimetres. Sure enough, I did! Although I hadn't been aware of having a mummy tummy or 'pooch' until that point, I suddenly felt self-conscious. The more I read, the more doomed I felt. According to a Pilates instructor interviewed by *Health* magazine, even getting out of bed without rolling onto my side could make it 'much worse'. Guilt and regret set in; for two years I'd been getting out of bed without executing a log roll. Within ten minutes, I went from feeling good about myself to losing all hope for the future of my abdomen.

I do not recommend you do what I did and google diastasis recti without a clear purpose. Unless you have perfect abs, it is likely to make you feel considerably worse about yourself – and, possibly, for no good reason. Remember that the fitness and physiotherapy sectors are industries, and they want people to buy their services; in my case, the blogs and articles I read managed to create a problem in order to provide a solution.

Dr Elwin Mommers, a Dutch academic with a PhD in abdominal wall repair, collaborated with physiotherapists to review the literature on diastasis recti in 2017. He came to two conclusions: that there is no research to show that physiotherapy closes the gap when your muscles are resting (which is when diastasis recti is, technically, defined), and that having a gap is not necessarily a bad thing. There is also no evidence to suggest that it leads to hernias, he says. For a small minority with a gap of at least 10 centimetres, the separation can seriously affect your quality of life, in which case surgery is an option – although Mommers cautions that surgery is only a cosmetic fix. If you are stable, don't have persistent back pain, if the connective tissue in between your abdominal muscles is firm and strong, and if it's not affecting your self-esteem, then you shouldn't need to worry about a mild tummy gap at all.

What Mommers did find was that physiotherapy can help reduce the gap by building up the muscles' bulk. Physiotherapy may also treat the symptoms of a tummy gap, he said – the mummy tummy, the instability, related pelvic floor dysfunction, pain and doming, for instance. Research has shown that diastasis recti and pelvic floor dysfunction often co-occur, so it's likely that, if you do see a physiotherapist for either of these, they will investigate the other and, if they find any weakness, address the two things together.

Sydney physiotherapist Antony Lo is another person who questions our obsession with diastasis recti. He even proposes that we see it as a natural adaptation to having had a baby inside you. 'You don't say to a dancer who can put their leg behind their head that they're injured. Calling it a "pooch" or a "mummy tummy" could be demonising something that doesn't need demonising,' he says. 'It's fine to make somebody like their tummy, but not to make them *not* like their tummy.'

A lot of women do find, however, that the abdominal weakness and separation affects them; beyond any physical symptoms, it can be a honey pot for anxiety and low self-esteem (although I can't say whether the anxiety fuels the semi-hysterical blog posts and articles online, or vice-versa).

While I don't recommend blindly googling it, I do, however, recommend you look up the blogs written by Wendy Powell at MUTU System on the subject. It's not the gap itself that's the problem, she writes, but the indication that something inside you isn't working right; she believes that diastasis is a symptom of a core not functioning optimally. The separation itself is not an issue, she explains, unless it causes your tummy to stick out, contributes to a weak and unstable core, if your back hurts, or if your pelvic floor doesn't work as it should.

How to test your tummy – and why our focus on 'the gap' is misleading

Most physios recommend you lie on your back with your knees bent and feet on the floor. Curl your head and neck up and probe the centre line of your belly. Can you feel the muscles engaging on either side? If so, how many fingers can you get between them? One or two fingers' widths is not usually considered a problem; more than that could be. But as important as the gap (if not more so) is actually the tension in the midline, according to physios. Contract your abs again and see how firm the tissue in between the muscles is. How far do your fingers sink in? If your midline feels firm like the end of your nose, your connective tissue is pretty strong; if it feels soft like your cheek, then it likely needs some work.

How to strengthen your tummy

The internet is full of articles and advice on how to 'close the gap', because that's what physiotherapy has traditionally focused on. On the internet, meanwhile, diastasis recti has become a sort of bogeyman and fall guy for when the problem is excess abdominal fat. But new research by the leading Canadian physiotherapist Diane Lee suggests that our focus on the gap is misguided. Diane believes that instead we should focus on increasing the tension in the tissue that connects the muscles – and postnatal health experts in the UK such as Wendy agree.

Physiotherapists recommend you take a whole-body approach to resolving symptoms, and that the first thing you should consider is your posture. The root cause of a gap is often your core not functioning as it should. Once you've worked on your posture (see page 243), you need to recruit and strengthen the deep muscles, which means starting with the transverse abdominus (or TVA) and obliques, the ones that hug you like a corset. (You should be working to strengthen your pelvic floor at the same time because it's all one system.) The breathing exercise on page 156, where you contract your pelvic floor, can achieve this and should be your starting point; simultaneously engage your deep abdominals, drawing your stomach in towards your spine, hold, then release as you inhale. Addressing these two things alone – your deep muscles and your posture – can have a big impact on your shape, but it can also directly affect your abdominal and pelvic floor function and benefit your body in the long term by redressing bad habits and building a solid base for the future.

Once you've established good posture and core engagement, you can do more core exercises, such as toe taps and single leg stretches. You can also do lunges and squats, which work the deep abdominals as well as the gluteus muscles (your bum) and hip stabilisers. Just avoid any exercises that cause your stomach to dome; whilst occasional, accidental doming isn't going to do any damage, it won't do any good either (see page 243) so you should stop and rest or modify an exercise if it happens. Increase the intensity of your core strength exercises as you get stronger but stay within the bounds of feeling comfortable and in control; good postnatal core-strength workouts should include exercises that load the tissue safely. If you do an exercise class like yoga, barre or Pilates, tell the instructor if you have some weakness or separation from the birth.

Advocates of massage therapy believe that abdominal muscles can fail to knit back together because of tight spots in the muscles or connective tissue in between. Tanya James, a massage therapist who runs Mother Massage in the UK, suggests you get to know your own tummy; feel for the rectus abdominus muscles and massage any tight or tender spots until the tenderness subsides. Lying down, you can try tilting your pelvis to arch your back and slowly travel up the abdominal muscle with your fingers applying pressure, one side at a time. Often, she says, by simply releasing areas of tightness you can restore function to the muscles and allow them to come back together.

Kate Walsh on 'doming':
'Think of a zip and being unable to close it after a big meal

because your tummy is bulging through it. Increased abdominal pressure can overwhelm abs that have been weakened by pregnancy and delivery so that you bulge out through the zip, hence the doming. It is an indicator that your muscle synergy is being overwhelmed by the abdominal pressure so, when it starts, you should rest and try again, or modify your activity. The eventual goal is to be able to go further and do more without doming. Some women will take more time to progress than others: some will have no gap ultimately; some will have a 2-centimetre gap with firm resistance and good function; others may have a 3-centimetre gap that's less firm but with good function, and others may not be able to reach that. A functional strong "corset" is the goal; the level at which that is achieved will be different for all women, in line with their lifestyle and expectations. This can be where the challenge lies, too, in managing your expectations!'

Breathing

Many of us know to breathe into our bellies rather than our shoulders or upper chest, which can create tension, but beyond that we don't tend to think about it. There is a proven link between how we breathe and rates of back pain and pelvic floor issues, however. With your diaphragm as the top of your pressurised cylinder, and your pelvic floor as the bottom, they are always working together. Your pelvic floor contracts when you breathe out, for example, so a forced expiration can lead to a stronger pelvic floor contraction. Breathing into your tummy, meanwhile, relaxes your pelvic floor (and if someone can't locate their pelvic floor muscles, getting them to breathe into their tummy and then contract on the exhale is one of the easiest ways to bring it to life).

In general, physios recommend that you aim for your chest, ribcage and abdomen to all expand evenly; no one of these should be more obvious than the other. If you find you're breathing too much into your chest or that your belly balloons out without your ribcage moving much, try to correct that; take a deep breath and focus on moving your lower ribcage and belly out and in together, then practise.

Umbilical hernia

Tanya James had three children in quick succession and years later found she was struggling to control her bladder. 'My God, I thought, what's happening? I wasn't quite fifty, and I was already beginning to wet myself,' she recalls. She also developed a bulge at her belly button. Having had cysts else-where in the past, she went to the doctor about what she thought was another one. 'Oh yes, that's definitely a cyst,' the doctor said. But it wasn't. It was an umbilical hernia, when a bit of fatty tissue or bowel pokes though a weak spot in the abdominal wall. Various health websites, including the NHS, give the impression that surgery is the only treatment option for this. In severe cases, such as when it's disrupting blood supply or creating a blockage, surgery will probably be necessary – but if yours is asymptomatic, like Tanya's, you should be able to manage it with exercises to strengthen your core, good alignment and breathing, and by eating a healthy, high-fibre diet.

Physiotherapist Antony Lo argues that we pile unneces-sary guilt on new mums for simply doing what they have to do: lifting more than a certain weight, not breath-ing 'correctly', letting go of our posture, or just rushing about like mad when we should be practising 'mindful' parenting:

'Stop making women feel bad about doing things. It's a myth that every time you see the linea alba distend it's a bad thing. Bending over and picking up something like a car seat is low pressure in terms of what those tissues are capable of. I've seen my wife give birth three times – now that's pressure. People say you're making it worse whenever you get that doming, but it's just a bit of distention; sure, you should try to limit it, but think of it like a balloon – we don't get upset when the balloon stretches – it's meant to stretch – but we get upset if someone stretches it to the point that it'll burst. If you lift a car seat, it's the way you lift it that's more important than the lifting itself.

'We should be training people to cope with normal everyday activities instead of restricting people and making them weaker, which actually increases their risk of injury because now they're not strong enough.'

17

Musculoskeletal Pain

Breastfeeding is a common culprit when it comes to post-natal musculoskeletal problems and pain. Tom Austen is an osteopath and father of three boys who specialises in treating babies, pregnant women and new mums. When a woman comes to see him at his clinic in Chester, he takes a detailed history and then goes from head to toe, looking at how everything in the body moves and how everything feels. The most common problems, he says, stem from the shoulders due to bad posture in the hours you spend breastfeeding and walking around with engorged breasts. 'Some women get paranoid about having a hump because the breast tissue is so heavy – it weighs down on the junction between your upper back and your neck so you feel that your shape is different,' he explains.

When breastfeeding, try to think about your posture from the start to avert future problems. Try to feed your baby evenly on both sides, he advises; it's good for your body, and it's good for the baby as well. Raise the baby on your lap if it helps to stop you stooping, or raise your knees by putting something underneath your feet. You could also put a cushion in the small of your back and use a chair with arms to give more support. Once the baby is feeding, try to sit back and relax your shoulders; it's very easy for tension to build up otherwise. Take a similar approach to posture when changing the baby – physios recommend that the changing mat be high enough for you to keep your head up and back straight while you're using it.

Another reason to look out for your posture while breast-feeding is relaxin, the hormone that loosens your ligaments in preparation for birth and remains elevated in your body until you've finished breastfeeding. If you have any structural weaknesses in your body, these can be exacerbated by relaxin – and bad posture is going to make them worse. Very often, Tom says, you see muscle fatigue in postpartum women; their muscles are having to work even harder than usual to support the joints because the ligaments are still quite wobbly. While you are breastfeeding, remember that your body will be less forgiving than usual, and you'll be more prone to injury, so avoid putting pressure on joints wherever possible (for more on posture, see page 243).

Another common problem is the pain we get (often in our necks and lower backs) from constantly hitching our hips and shoulders up to support our children. The number of tasks a mother can do at once – for example, hold and comfort a child, stir porridge, make a phone call and clear toys from beneath her feet, all at once – is astonishing. But it's also in part why our bodies tend to suffer. If you're at the stage where your children and their gear require a lot of hefting and hitching, try to use both hips, arms and shoulders alternately to prevent stiffness and soreness.

Pelvic girdle pain

Previously called symphysis pubis dysfunction (SPD), pelvic girdle pain comes from either the front of the pelvis, where your pubic bone is, or at the back where your pelvis connects to the spine on both sides with the sacroiliac joints. While it starts in the pelvis, it often radiates to the hips or thighs. It usually goes away within four months of giving birth, but for one in five women who had it during pregnancy, it continues for years. The exact causes are not well understood, but physiotherapy and manual therapy like osteopathy can help, as can lifestyle changes, for example, getting help with your share of the household chores (activities like hoovering, mopping, raking up leaves or shovelling snow are all linked to lower back pain), or avoiding sitting down for too long. The Royal College of Obstetricians and Gynaecologists say that, while it's common, it's not something women should put up with – so if your pain persists, get a referral (or refer yourself) to a physiotherapist, osteopath or chiropractor who specialises in pelvic girdle pain. (In the Resources section, you'll find a link to a helpful pamphlet published by the Royal College of Obstetricians and Gynaecologists on managing pelvic girdle pain as well as other common conditions during and after pregnancy.)

De Quervain syndrome (Mother's wrist)

Harriet's baby loved it when she held her under the arms and bounced her up and down. Harriet loved it too, until she developed excruciating pain in her arms and wrists. 'I couldn't even lift the kettle – and I needed a lot of tea,' she recalls. Rather than stop whatever she was doing whenever the pain occurred, she would power on through, channelling her inner lion: 'I was like, "Roar, my arms will learn." But they were actually pleading with me, saying "stop, we're breaking".' Eventually, Harriet went to see a doctor who told her to lift her baby less. 'Clearly, he had never had to look after a baby on his own,' she said. It took around six months for the problem to resolve, but she believes that if she had known to be more careful when it first appeared, it would never have become so bad.

Thumb and wrist pain in pregnant women and new mums is called De Quervain's tenosynovitis, or mother's wrist. It's not fully understood but it's thought that hormone changes, excess fluid in the body and the extra pressure we put on our hands and wrists with a new baby can irritate the tendons and their sheathes that travel down your wrists and into your thumbs, causing inflammation. The pain can start during pregnancy, when your levels of the hormone relaxin are unusually high, or it can come on afterwards.

A simple test known as the Finkelstein's test can diagnose it. Bend your thumb across your palm, curl your fingers down over your thumb, then bend your wrist towards your little finger. If this is painful down your wrist around the base of your thumb, it's likely to be Quervain's tenosynovitis.

The best advice is to stop doing whatever causes the pain wherever you can. Immobilising your thumb and wrist with a splint or brace can help to rest the tendons. And you should avoid repetitive movements, particularly with your thumb; your tendons need to rest in order to get better. You can take ibuprofen for the pain and apply ice to the affected wrist. Doctors say that symptoms should improve within four to six weeks – a long time to be in pain whenever you need to lift your baby – but if they don't ease you should go back because there are more things doctors can recommend, including injections of corticosteroids to reduce the inflammation.

Feet

If you're wondering why your shoes are tighter than before, it's because your feet may now be bigger. On average, a woman puts on nearly two stone during pregnancy. This extra weight on her feet, combined with the elasticity hormone, relaxin, can cause the arches to drop, so the feet get longer. The gold-medal-winning 10,000-metre runner Jo Pavey (see Chapter 18) found that just one of her feet got longer during pregnancy when the ligaments weakened, changing the mechanics of her foot. Years later, she was still wearing a bigger shoe on her left foot.

Rather than condemn yourself to buying double the shoes for the rest of your life, if one of your arches drops (or if both of them drop), there is a good chance that you can reverse it by doing exercises that strengthen the muscles underneath your foot. The reasons for doing so go beyond the practicalities of buying new shoes; flat feet can have a knock-on effect on your knees, hips and lower back. If your arches collapse, your knees will usually move inwards a little, putting more pressure on the inside of the knees and even changing the angle of your hipbones. If you have weak or tight spots in the lower back, hips or pelvis, it can exacerbate these issues, or it can predispose you to problems further down the line, such as your joints wearing out more quickly than they should. If you want to know how to fix your flat feet, the website fixflatfeet.com, set up by California-based physical therapist James Speck, is a good place to start.

18

Exercise

'If the body be feeble, the mind will not be strong.'

Thomas Jefferson

Along with sleep, exercise is considered one of nature's panaceas, good for balancing hormones, preventing disease and strengthening our immune systems. But it is about far more than just physical health or 'getting fit'; it can revive your sense of place in the world, release creativity, and provide you with a hit of endorphins that boost your mood and change how you feel about your life. But where do you start? Do whatever makes you happy, most would say. But what if the thing that makes you happy is incompatible with your body? What if all you want to do is cross-fit or running, and you have an injury that makes any sort of exertion a misery? The good news is that you probably don't need to give up on your favourite form of exercise; it might just take some time and hard work before you get there. 'I have had powerlifters with prolapses, OASIs, all sorts of pelvic floor dysfunctions, who have managed to retrain so they can engage their pelvic floor in a safe way, whilst training in exactly the way they want to,' said Kate Walsh. 'So I do think that you can usually achieve more than you think you can.' Start slowly, continue to work on your core and pelvic floor strength, and build up the intensity and endurance consistently and systematically.

The basics of postpartum exercise

Ideally, everyone would see a pelvic health physiotherapist as they're getting back into exercise, but that's not always feasible. So the question we need an answer to is this: if you want to exercise and feel ready for more than breathing and squeezing, how can you judge for yourself what's safe, but also challenging enough to make a difference to your strength and fitness? Here are a few words of advice, drawn from a number of physiotherapists:

Watch your core – It's important to get your core muscles – diaphragm, spinal muscles, abdominals and pelvic floor – working well before doing anything else (see page 242). Be careful doing exercises that increase the pressure in your abdomen, such as a plank or sit-ups (see page 275). If the corset of muscles and tissue around your abdomen is weak, any pressure you exert on your abdomen may overwhelm the muscles and lead to doming. Lots of exercises, such as squats and lunges, can strengthen the core without overwhelming the abs like crunches and sit-ups do, so stick to these instead. (In fact, sit-ups aren't considered great for anybody; even the US armed forces is currently phasing them out.) Before doing anything high-impact like running you should check your pelvic floor strength and, if necessary, work on it first.

Adapt – Any exercise can be adapted to fit your personal level of core strength, so there's no need to push it beyond what feels right. Modify whatever you want to do, so that you build up your strength and endurance safely. If you do this, you may soon find you don't need the modification.

Relaxin – If you're still breastfeeding, you have higher levels of relaxin than normal, which leaves you more prone to injury. Don't push your body as far as you would have done before pregnancy until you've stopped breastfeeding and your muscles and ligaments feel stable again.

Sleep – Not getting much sleep is another reason to be more careful than usual; being sleep-deprived doubles your risk of injury, according to sleep scientist Matthew Walker.

Breastfeeding – You probably want to exercise after a feed or pumping so that your breasts are empty. Research suggests that moderate exercise does not generally impact a woman's milk supply. Particularly strenuous exercise can temporarily cause higher levels of lactic acid in your milk – but all this may do is occasionally make your baby fussier at the breast immediately afterwards, when lactic acid levels are still high.

> **Julie Wiebe, *personal trainer.***
> 'The overarching rules I set for my patients are if you lose your breath or your alignment (form) during the activity, it is too challenging.'

Walking

Walking is one of the most undervalued forms of exercise, and it's perfect if you have a baby or small children. If your pelvic floor feels strong enough, put the baby in a sling, or use a pushchair if not, and head out for a brisk walk. Putting one foot in front of the other not only improves your physical health on all fronts, it also boosts your creativity and mental health. As the philosopher Friedrich Nietzsche wrote in 1889: 'All truly great thoughts are conceived by walking.' It's low-impact, you can do it for longer than running, and babies love it too. If you get to a hill and you're pushing a pram, try to keep your ribs stacked above your pelvis and your body close to the pram. Your glutes – your bum muscles – should be the ones powering you up the hill, but sometimes these muscles need a little activation. Look up the exercise known as a clamshell to help awaken yours. Likewise, if you're pushing a pram downhill, physios recommend you resist the temptation to lean back; stay close to the pram, keep your ribs above your pelvis, and use your glutes to slow you down.

Pilates and yoga

Pilates, yoga, barre or any other core strength and stability workout that doesn't involve impact is ideal for when you're feeling a bit out of joint and your core is still recovering from childbirth. You can also try doing it with a baby lying on your mat. If you do a class, tell the instructor if you have any weaknesses or concerns, listen to your body, and adapt exercises that feel too hard. Be judicious about who you take advice from; not all pre- and postnatal Pilates or yoga classes will include exercises that are right for your body, so learn to trust what it's telling you and see a physiotherapist if something is niggling you. There are also lots of free classes on YouTube to try.

Mum and baby classes

There is an extraordinary array of mum and baby exercise classes around, particularly if you live in a city where you can choose anything from fusion ballet and Pilates classes to salsa. Classes like this also provide an opportunity to socialise. If you prefer to sweat and socialise separately, however, there are a growing number of online classes (particularly since the coronavirus pandemic). If they involve high-impact exercises or targeted abdominal work, be sensible; if something brings on symptoms (for example, signs of urinary or faecal incontinence), or you find you're struggling to keep your body in alignment (such as getting doming in your tummy), adapt the exercise or stop. If everything feels good, you're probably fine; but if something doesn't feel right somehow, see a physiotherapist for an assessment.

Swimming

Swimming is low impact and the water provides resistance, working your heart and lungs without putting pressure on your joints. You might also find postnatal water aerobics classes. The NHS recommends you wait until a week after any bleeding has finished, and obviously until any stitches have healed. If you have any weakness or separation in your abdominal muscles, wear goggles so that you're not arching your back and flaring out your ribcage to keep your head above water; physios say that your spine should be in a neutral position as you swim to keep everything in alignment.

Running

When to start running postpartum, like all impact sports, is a controversial subject amongst physiotherapists and fitness professionals. Some women, like Jasmin Paris (see page 277), feel ready to start jogging again within a few weeks, but they are in the minority. At the other end of the spectrum, if you have damaged your core and pelvic floor, it may take you a year or more of strength training to feel stable enough (see page 273).

UK guidelines – three to six months

In 2019, three British physiotherapists developed new guidelines that recommend women wait at least three to six months before running until the pelvis is fully healed. Few women feel stable enough in their pelvis to start running at six weeks, the researchers say, and too often women run whilst leaking, covering their symptoms by wearing a pad or black leggings; by doing so, they make things worse for themselves. 'The bugbear for all of us clinicians is that awful six-week green light to go ahead and pretty much do what you want – which couldn't be more untrue,' said Emma Brockwell, one of three physiotherapists behind the guidelines.

Their report, 'Returning to running postnatal', is written for health professionals but is available online and contains lots of good information. They advise that you see a women's health physio before returning to any form of high-impact exercise, running included, and state that you are not ready to run if you experience any of the following:

- Urinary leakage
- Faecal incontinence or obstruction

- Heaviness in the vagina
- Pain during sex
- Doming, if you have diastasis recti
- Pelvic pain.

If you're clear of these symptoms in normal postpartum life, you can try hopping, jumping forwards, running on the spot, walking for half an hour, and standing on one leg. If doing so throws up problems, again, you're probably not ready to run. It's recommended that you see a pelvic health physiotherapist who will do a vaginal exam to assess the strength of your muscles and consider how well the connective tissues have recovered.

By taking your time now, physios urge, you'll be future-proofing your ability to exercise later. But if you're really desperate to return to running sooner than recommended, they suggest that you consider running on an incline – either a treadmill or a hill – which decreases the impact on your abdomen and pelvic floor, or using an elliptical trainer, which is low-impact but provides a similar workout. And continue with your core and pelvic floor muscle training at the same time. If you don't show any of the above symptoms whilst hopping, jumping, running on the spot and walking, the guidelines say that you should be ready to resume running.

The bespoke approach

Antony Lo, the Australian physiotherapist mentioned earlier, challenges the assumption that by running before you have fully rehabilitated your pelvic floor you will be 'making things worse'. Most advice is too conservative, he says, and women's bodies can take more than we commonly assume before further damage occurs; you can, of course, make things worse by overloading the abdomen or pelvic floor, he says, but running and stopping to rest whenever you feel symptoms coming on is unlikely to do further harm (see Anna's story, page 331).

Antony believes that pelvic floor muscle rehabilitation can and should be done alongside whatever sport you choose, running included, and it can even help your pelvic floor recovery by improving the muscles' functionality, putting into practice the isolated strength training you've been doing. If it's running you want to get back to, you may have to run uphill and walk downhill to reduce the impact on your pelvic floor, run on grass, and stop before becoming symptomatic. Although Antony doesn't advise continuing to run after symptoms appear, he acknowledges that it's a woman's choice to do so.

Whatever you decide to do, listen carefully to your body and act accordingly. If in any doubt, make an appointment with a pelvic health physiotherapist. But remember that a good physio should ask what you want to achieve and then help you get there – not dictate to you what you must and must not do.

Angela Cross, a mother of three, had a minor vaginal prolapse after her first baby and was told she would never run again. She can now squat-lift 75 kilogrammes and run for 40 minutes without symptoms, despite having had two more children:

'I went to see a sports physio who specialises in women's health. When I first went to him, I couldn't run more than 30 seconds without leaking, no matter how slowly I ran; it didn't help if I went to the bathroom and left the house straightaway. He

convinced me to give him a year; there were parts of the training I wouldn't enjoy, he warned, but I'd get there.

'At first, I had to run on grass until I started having symptoms, then I would stop, walk, rest, and start again. I was so slow, I felt like a geriatric who'd been let out of the nursing home, and I'd be lucky if I got to 20 or 30 seconds. This isn't going to work, I thought. But, gradually, it did. He encouraged me to start CrossFit at the same time. The gym was briefed on my injuries and they worked out what I couldn't do – which was basically anything that caused me to have symptoms. As I understood it, I needed to bulk up down there; there was no real resistance in the Pilates I'd been doing, so it would only get me to a certain level and not necessarily get me back to running. Lifting weights and doing CrossFit exercises with a focus on functional fitness, would be good for my injuries, he said.

'My body – and particularly my core – got stronger and I learned to run again. I went from being able to run for 30 seconds to being able to run for 90 seconds, then to ten minutes, then to 20 minutes... At that point, he said I had to get off the grass. Now, I can just run out of my house and go for 40 minutes without any symptoms.

'For someone who considers themselves a runner, being told you can't run is bigger news than the person delivering it realises. Exercise becomes a part of who you are when you've been doing it for several years. A part of me never completely accepted I wouldn't be able to run again, and it's lovely to have that alone time as a mother; I'm outdoors, doing something that I love. And I've gone from being told I couldn't lift anything more than 10 kilos to squatting and lifting 75 kilos and doing as many box jumps as I like. Throughout all of this, I've been seeing my women's health physio to make sure *the lifting and running weren't making my injuries worse. At the end of last year, she said that all my injuries were in the best shape they've ever been, and that if I continue like this, I won't need surgery in my lifetime.'*

Postnatal exercise and the culture of fear

When my son was about 18 months old and putting him to bed could be a long and tedious process, I would often use the time while he settled to quietly do a Pilates plank on the floor, lying flat like a board raised up on my elbows and toes. When I later learned about diastasis recti, and discovered a three centimetre or so gap between my abdominal muscles, I panicked. Planks are dangerous for anyone with a diastasis, I read, and can make it worse. Likewise, trying to run before you're ready can damage your pelvic floor, physios and fitness professionals said. With my well-intentioned exercising, had I been doing more harm than good?

I unwittingly became a victim of what some physios call the 'culture of fear' surrounding postnatal health. The Californian physiotherapist Julie Wiebe once implored her colleagues to watch their language so as not to add to it. In a long Facebook post, she explained that her patients with diastasis were feeling betrayed and paralysed with fear by the contradictory advice: that they should do exercises like the plank for their abs, but that now they were postnatal, they should never do a plank or abdominal work again. 'Do we really mean never do a plank again? Or do we mean let's restore abdominal function and fascial density and find exercises you can do, which absolutely may one day include a plank?' Julie asked.

In response to her question, the acclaimed pelvic floor expert and former US military captain Ramona Horton backed her up. Ramona even went a step further, dismissing the notion that women with diastasis can never do planks as 'pure conjecture and a load of balderdash'. She likened it to saying that women shouldn't do head stands for fear that their stomach could pop out of their throat. As long as a woman has good control of her deep abdominal muscles and is not holding her breath or exhaling forcefully, she has absolutely no reason to avoid planks, Ramona wrote.

Part of the problem is that we don't have the level of information we need to make safe and confident choices. 'If we are truly about empowering people, we cannot continue patronising them', says Antony Lo. 'We need to leave our clients thinking they're strong, capable, adaptable and resilient, as opposed to thinking that they're weak, inflexible, fragile – all the adjectives that people hate.'

In every other realm of rehabilitation, Antony says, we gradually increase the load on a muscle until it does whatever you need it to again. When it comes to women's postnatal health, however, the blanket – and, he argues, paternalistic – advice is to avoid loading the muscles – don't lift anything heavy, don't do any impact sport, don't do abdominal work, and don't load your pelvic floor unnecessarily; walk, swim and do yoga, Pilates and pelvic floor squeezes instead. But how can we claim to be feminists if we're controlling what women can and can't do with their bodies?

It all comes down to safety – *do no harm* is one of the founding principles of modern medicine – and psychology. Physios worry that, if they dilute their advice to make it less stringent, women might ignore it altogether and, as a result, end up doing harm. But equally, are we not capable of digesting more complex advice and taking informed decisions alongside health professionals about what's safe and what's not?

A lot of physios advise that you listen to your body – it knows best. But how we feel about our bodies is influenced by what we believe, as I discovered when I started googling diastasis recti. The bottom line is that everyone is different, and complex issues require an individualised, holistic approach that is based on a good understanding of sound scientific principles. If you're working out all of this alone, try to make choices without being ruled by anxiety and generic – sometimes fear-mongering – advice.

World Champion fell-runner and mother of two Jasmin Paris smashed expectations – as well as the UK's most gruelling race record – shortly after the birth of her first child.

The British fell-running champion Jasmin Paris had an inkling of what childbirth could do to your body, but she wanted to be a mother more than she wanted to be a runner, so she was willing to risk it. She ran her last race ten days before her daughter was born and, despite her baby being breech, had a good delivery, her pelvic floor felt fine, and – as proof that everyone's body is different – she started walking and jogging three weeks afterwards. 'It's like a drug, a positive drug, and I didn't lose that feeling of wanting to get out and do it,' she says. Her biggest challenge was time. Early mornings, 6 a.m. to 8 a.m., she would run in the hills and feel like herself. It's what kept her sane, she reflects, two years later. Another training strategy was to do hill reps and intervals while her daughter slept, in clear view, in her buggy.

Five months after the birth, Jasmin stood on the start-line of her first race as a mother – nine and a half miles across the Mourne Mountains, whose precipitous granite peaks inspired C.S. Lewis' Narnia. Jasmin felt unprepared, trepidatious. The weather was awful: thick fog. And the race was linear, point-to-point, which meant no ducking out halfway. Would her baby be crying for milk whilst she was out on the course, she wondered? To Jasmin's surprise, the race went well – so well that she was the first woman home, and in good time to feed her daughter. Her next race was less triumphant; it was the day after her daughter's vaccinations, and Jasmin had been up most of the night. But after that came a string of successes. Could motherhood have improved her running, friends and commentators started to ask? She regained her title as British Champion and, hankering after a new challenge, she did something 'crazy' by entering the 268-mile Spine race, one of the toughest ultra-marathons in Europe that crosses the Pennine Way in mid-January.

Her 6 a.m. starts shifted to 5 a.m. in order to fit in training before work. Her coach told her to wear a weight vest, but carrying a baby had the same effect. Jasmin intended to wean her daughter before the race, but it didn't happen because her daughter got sick – so Jasmin was still breastfeeding when it came about.

Competitors in the Spine race expect blizzards, heavy rain, waist-deep snow, 50mph gales and severe wind chill. At checkpoints along the way, most just refuel and catnap, but Jasmin also had to express milk to stop her boobs becoming uncomfortable. By the end of the race, the thought of getting back to her family drove her on, but hallucinations threatened to derail her – she saw animals emerging from rocks and even forgot where she was.

She was out racing for 83 hours and 12 minutes in total. This sounds like a very long time, until you know that she was out on the course for 12 hours fewer than any other competitor in the race's history. Jasmin smashed all previous course

*records, men's included, and in doing so made running – and
mothering – history.*

*She's not sure whether motherhood has helped her
running, but definitely thinks it helped her to go without
sleep, which played a hand in the Spine race, when she slept
for just three hours in three and a half days.*

Could childbirth improve athletic performance?

Paris's performance has led experts to question whether
the improved strength and endurance of some women after
they become mums could have something to do with childbirth. Firstly, the ribcage expands during pregnancy, which
might allow endurance athletes to take in more air. Secondly,
and perhaps more importantly, are the changes to the cardiovascular system – your heart and blood vessels. During
pregnancy, the chambers of your heart get larger to allow for
more blood to flow through. Theoretically, this makes the
heart more efficient at getting oxygen to the muscles, so it
can work more comfortably.

Jo Pavey, a British long-distance runner, made history
in 2014 when, at the age of 40, she won the 10,000 metres at
the World Championships in Zurich, just ten months after
having her second child. Jo, who wrote the book *This Mum
Runs*, has spoken about the many challenges of getting back
into sport after having children, but also found two key hormonal benefits: her body was better at regulating blood sugar
after having children, and her menstrual cycles were easier
to handle. 'Your body definitely seems to calm down once
you've reproduced,' she told the *Guardian* in 2014. Whether
a woman's pain threshold is higher after childbirth is hard to
prove because pain is subjective, but that's another possibility.

19

Diet and Weight

Once you've made it through the first six weeks, much of your body's major healing is complete, but your nutrient stocks will still be low, and your energy needs still higher than usual, with the exertions of caring for a baby as well as making milk if you are breastfeeding (and, possibly, looking after other children). This is when the long-term exhaustion and depletion can kick in and, if you're not careful, you become a sleep-starved zombie with the emotional resilience of a toddler.

Postnatal depletion

Oscar Serrallach is a doctor who moved from a busy Australian town to pursue a life of self-sufficiency in rural New South Wales. He and his wife had three children and, while these should have been the happiest of times, Serrallach watched his wife become more miserable and drained with each one. They hit crisis point soon after their third child was born. Her memory and concentration were shot, she felt constantly overwhelmed and enveloped by fog, had lost her confidence, felt isolated, and even struggled to take care of herself fully. 'She was extremely fatigued, suffered anxiety, felt her sleep was superficial at best, and had a deep fear that she was never going to recover,' Oscar writes in his book, *The Postnatal Depletion Cure.*

Desperate to help, Oscar started studying his patients and quickly found that his wife's condition was far from rare. So many mothers felt just like her and seemed to have given up hope of ever recovering. Oscar concluded that if a new mother isn't allowed to fully recover from pregnancy and birth, then the after-effects can plague her for years. He eventually labelled his wife's syndrome Postnatal Depletion and devised a treatment plan for her and the millions of other women who were suffering in the same way. It takes a multi-pronged approach: emotional support, dietary changes, vitamin and mineral support, herbal supplements, alternative therapies, restorative yoga, breathing and meditation, and better sleep. When you feel broken and don't have enough hours in the day to shower let alone meditate, this might sound like an unlikely solution to your fatigue. But one of the core pillars of his practice, nutrition, should be within everyone's grasp. In recognition of this, the NHS gives women receiving certain benefits who are pregnant or have a child up to the age of one free vitamins for the mother, as well as vouchers to spend on milk, fresh and frozen fruit and vegetables and formula for the child; the vouchers for the child continue until the age of four.

In terms of your diet, to replace what you've lost – and, if you're breastfeeding, continue to lose – experts like Oscar Serrallach and Lily Nichols largely agree: you need to eat a diet that is high in nutrients, and that means one that is higher in fats than you might be used to, with moderately high levels of protein and lower levels of carbohydrates (especially processed grains, which don't contain much in terms of nutrients) – although they caution that your diet shouldn't be strictly low-carb when you're postpartum, unless you're confident that it's not affecting your energy levels and milk supply.

How to eat a nutrient-rich diet

Lily Nichols is a crusading food detective known for debunking diet myths and exposing poorly evidenced guidelines. She is passionate about the postnatal period and dedicates a long chapter to it in her book, *Real Food for Pregnancy*. When I interviewed her, she was nine months postpartum and, like me, living her subject area, navigating the peaks and troughs of motherhood with an element of detached interest and a notebook at the ready. The problem with a diet high in carbs, she explains, is that it's often at the expense of foods that provide the most nutrients; carb consumption is inversely linked to a person's micronutrient intake, especially if those carbohydrates are from refined or processed sources. In the US, an estimated 85 per cent of carbohydrates are consumed from processed foods and sugar. She recommends we see carbs (such as white potatoes, rice and pasta) as condiments, rather than the mainstays of our diet, and instead eat a greater proportion and variety of vegetables in their place, in order to raise our nutrient intake (see page 291, for the pillars of postnatal nutrition).

Supplements for depletion

A good postnatal supplement should contain the basics in terms of your nutrient needs. If you want to be more specific, however, Oscar Serrallach recommends the following:

- Iron Bisglycinate – 15–24 milligrams for six weeks if you think you have low levels of iron.
- DHA fish oil or algae oil, 1 gram (or 1.5 grams if you're breastfeeding) daily for six weeks.
- 175 milligrams choline per day for six weeks, to help with concentration.
- Zinc picolinate or citrate, 25 milligrams per day with food for six weeks to help the brain and immune system.
- Magnesium for sleep and muscle relaxation, 150 milligrams once or twice per day – especially good before bed (and if you get restless legs, like me).

Eating for breastfeeding

One of the more compelling arguments for a pregnant woman or new mother to ditch the cake in favour of real foods is that breast milk is 'conditionally perfect', as the Boston nutritionist Miriam Erick writes. This means that your food choices can affect it, and a nutrient deficiency in you could be carried forwards into your milk. Don't take this to mean that formula may be better for your baby than breast-milk – your body has compensation mechanisms that mean your breastmilk will always be the healthiest thing you can give your child. But you can eat to super-charge it, as well as to ensure you don't deplete your own reserves while feeding your baby.

The most common deficiencies in breast milk in the West are vitamin D, iodine, iron and vitamin K. As a general guide, eat a wide variety of nutrient-rich foods, including plenty of healthy fat, iron, protein and leafy green vegetables to ensure your milk contains everything your baby needs;

most nutritionists will recommend you take a postnatal multivitamin as a safety net.

Vitamin D – A 2015 American study found that almost all exclusively breastfed babies were vitamin-D deficient if they weren't receiving a supplement. That's not because breast milk doesn't confer enough vitamin D; it's because most mums are vitamin-D deficient, so don't have enough to pass on. You can give your baby a supplement, or just take the supplement yourself to ensure they get enough.

Iodine – Iodine deficiency is common amongst pregnant women in the UK. Unlike in other countries, table salt in the UK is not usually iodised; instead, milk is our principal source of iodine. Dairy cows receive an iodine supplement, and therefore express relatively high levels in their milk – but not organic cows, who aren't supplemented in the same way, which is why organic milk contains lower amounts. To ensure your baby is getting enough iodine, seaweed (if you can find it) is the ultimate source, but you can also just eat plenty of fish and dairy.

Vitamin K – It's likely that your baby received an injection shortly after it was born, but it will need more. Formula contains more vitamin K than breastmilk and it's important that you have enough to prevent your milk becoming deficient. Kale is a great source of this, as are most green vegetables including spinach, sprouts and broccoli.

Iron – Globally, almost 40 per cent of pregnant women are anaemic, and childbirth can deplete your iron stores further. Because the symptoms of iron deficiency are similar to what we all associate with early motherhood – fatigue, an inability to concentrate, problems sleeping and headaches – it can get missed. Nutritionists warn that it's difficult to meet your iron needs when breastfeeding if you're not eating shellfish like oysters, clams and mussels, or organ meats like liver – but not all of us want to be eating liver (even though it's cheap) or shellfish (which is expensive). Spinach, red meat, beans, nuts and fortified cereals are good sources of iron. If you're vegetarian or vegan, it's recommended that you take a good-quality iron supplement that should contain additional nutrients to support absorption. There are lots of different types of iron, but research supports the use of ferrous bisglycinate, because it's relatively well absorbed and shouldn't cause constipation (as other types can).

Vitamin B12 – This essential vitamin is only available from animal sources – although foods like some cereals, plant-based milks and malt extract are fortified with vitamin B12. You don't need a lot of it, and if you eat animal products you're likely to get enough. If you are breastfeeding and you are a strict vegetarian or vegan, however, there's a greater chance that you're deficient, and that your baby could become so too; a recent literature review found that a quarter of mums were deficient in B12 across all three trimesters. And a 2015 article published in the *Journal of Nutrition* found that your B12 needs when pregnant or breastfeeding are around triple the current amount (2.8 micrograms) that's recommended. Based on this, if you're vegetarian or vegan and breastfeeding, you should be taking a supplement that provides at least 10 micrograms per day, which is also in line with the Vegan Society's recommendation.

Inflammation

Oscar Serrallach believes the key hallmark of postnatal depletion – when women become 'zombie-like, diaper-changing,
milking machines', as he puts it – is inflammation. Anyone
who's been pregnant knows that inflammation of tissues in
the body is an unavoidable – and perfectly normal – consequence of pregnancy. But too much of it can cause stress
and deplete your nutrient bank to the point that you end up
physically and mentally compromised, Oscar says.

There are proven links between inflammation in the
body and our mental health: a diet that is considered inflammatory – which has, for example, lots of red meat and refined
sugar – is linked to depression and other mental health disorders. Likewise, a diet low in inflammatories (see the list
below) can remedy depression, and one study even found it
as effective as many chemical antidepressants. To prove the
point, some doctors are now successfully treating depression
with anti-inflammatories alone. Not all depression is linked
to inflammation but, as new evidence emerges every year,
leading medical professionals – people who grew up thinking
there was a big red line between mental and physical health
– are coming around to the idea that inflammation is part
of the problem in all sorts of conditions in the human body.

As scientists discover more about the links between inflammation – dubbed the new frontier of medical science – and
mental health, the barriers that used to divide mental and
physical health are crumbling. While more traditional health
systems still embrace the notion of body and mind being one,
we in the West have developed a prejudice against it, and leading scientists and doctors are now urging us to reconsider it.

In January 2020, a young American psychiatrist called
Eric Achtyes published his study into the links between

inflammation and severe depression and suicidal behaviour in postnatal women. Inflammation, he said, is a normal part of pregnancy, but when the inflammatory response lasts longer or is more intense than normal, it can lead to worsening depression. Achtyes hopes that his findings will mean women are one day offered treatments specifically for 'inflammatory' postnatal depression. In the meantime, we can follow a diet that's shown to be good for our mental health.

Foods to avoid, which cause inflammation, include:

- refined carbohydrates, such as white bread and pastries
- deep-fried food
- sugar-sweetened drinks
- red meat (burgers, steaks) and processed meat (hot dogs, sausage)
- margarine, shortening and lard.

Foods to indulge in, which reduce inflammation, include:

- olive oil
- green leafy veg, such as spinach and kale
- nuts, like almonds and walnuts
- fatty fish, like salmon, mackerel, tuna and sardines
- fruits, such as strawberries, blueberries, cherries and oranges.

Do you really need expensive supplements?

Women have been giving birth to and nourishing healthy babies for millennia without taking pre- and postnatal vitamins. I think of my grandmother's generation, who raised their babies during the war and the long period of rationing that came afterwards. And of all of the strong, quick-witted men and women I met whilst in Turkana, northern Kenya, who were raised under the constant shadow of drought. I doubt any of us consume a 'perfect' diet, not that we even know what that is. And as soil and food quality around the world is declining, as experts claim, it's almost impossible to know exactly what we're consuming and what its nutritional value is.

Currently, the official UK advice is that women take 400 micrograms of folic acid each day, from before pregnancy up to 12 weeks, and 10 micrograms of vitamin D each day when pregnant and breastfeeding; otherwise, there is no need for a vitamin supplement in a well-nourished woman, the NHS says, and eating a balanced diet is the best way to ensure a healthy mother and child. So why supplement?

Nutritionists argue that supplements act as a safety net to combat gaps in a woman's diet. Postnatal vitamins range from the cheap packs you find in discount stores to the kind sold by specialist naturopaths that cost ten times as much – and choosing between them can be daunting. We tend to trust the brands with which we're best acquainted, but who's to say they're not spending most of their budgets on marketing rather than on the quality of their product?

Naturopaths argue that if you're taking the cheap ones, you may as well be eating Lego. The quality of a multivitamin relies mostly on how well the body absorbs it. Cheap multivitamins tend to contain vitamins derived from chemical compounds, they warn, which the body doesn't always absorb. The more expensive multivitamins, however, tend to have better 'bioavailability', often because the vitamins they contain are derived from food.

ConsumerLab, the American supplement industry

watchdog, backs up these concerns about cheap supplements. They recently found that over half of the mainstream multivitamins in the US contain either more or less of stated ingredients. Some were contaminated with other substances, including lead. And many do not get properly absorbed.

On the other hand, the ingredients of most multivitamins are simply commodity items; like sugar and coffee, they are raw materials, traded on a global market. As a 2009 *New York Times* article writes, 'every manufacturer has access to the same ingredients. For that reason, researchers and scientists say paying more for a name brand won't necessarily buy you better vitamins.'

With the amount of uncertainty surrounding this controversial subject, the one thing everyone agrees on is that there is no substitute for a healthy, balanced and varied diet. Beyond folic acid and vitamin D, which have enough evidence behind them for the government to recommend them, it's up to you what you choose in terms of supplements. Vitamins do, however, degrade over time, and need to be stored at or below room temperature, so get them from somewhere that restocks regularly and watch the expiry date.

Postpartum weight loss

Nutritionists and personal trainers use the phrase 'nine months on, nine months off', because they consider nine months a sensible timeframe for losing the baby weight you've spent the past nine months accumulating. Postpartum weight loss is, however, unpredictable and different for everyone; no matter how much you want to return to your pre-baby weight by nine months, your body may have other plans.

Straight after the birth, everyone loses weight at roughly the same rate, as they lose the placenta and amniotic fluid, and blood volume, uterus and other tissues contract. Beyond six weeks, it's more complicated. Breastfeeding devotees say that exclusive breastfeeding is nature's weight-loss remedy; you can expend up to 650 extra calories a day in the first six months, even if you're just lying on the sofa. And some breastfeeding women do lose their extra weight very easily. Breastfeeding can also be, however, a licence to gorge on crumpets and cake. The hormones you make stimulate appetite; breastfeeding women are usually ravenous and easily make up for the calorie deficit in snacks. And, although breastfeeding increases the number of calories you need, it also seems to encourage the body to hold on to fat reserves, particularly on the arms, and some women only drop their excess weight when they stop – as far as two years down the line.

Ultimately, it seems that your lifestyle and genetics will determine how and when you lose the extra weight, not whether you breastfeed or not. A 2004 study found that postpartum mums who breastfed and those that didn't lost weight at a similar rate (but those who breastfed lost fat less quickly). If you were overweight before pregnancy, or gained more than the recommended amount whilst pregnant, you may find the weight harder to lose; some women even put on weight after the first six weeks. Research shows that one in five women are still carrying an extra five kilos or more a year after the birth.

Real food diet

Before you go on any sort of radical diet, try cutting out the rubbish and eating just 'real food', as Lily Nichols calls it. The diet she proposes is lower in carbohydrates and higher in protein and fat that you might normally eat, based on the following principles:

1. Eat unprocessed, whole foods

Lily does not encourage clients to focus on weight loss for several months after the birth – she's a proponent of the nine months on, nine months off theory, and has seen plenty of clients unable to lose all their extra weight until they stop breastfeeding. Instead, your starting point should be to focus on eating nutrient-dense, real foods – so cut back on empty calories from sugars and fillers like cereals including wheat, maize, rice and oats, crackers and other processed foods. You'll need some carbs because your energy needs are so high, but they should be an add-on rather than the main event. By eating mostly vegetables, meat, fish, eggs, dairy, nuts, seeds, legumes and fruit with plenty of fat and protein, you'll stabilise your blood sugar level and maximise nutrient intake. Lily knows what it's like to gorge on biscuits when your child finally goes down for the nap they've been fighting all afternoon. Try to find replacements for the sugary, nutrient-poor foods that sneak in at times like that – because if you can manage to eat more nutrient-dense food, Lily says, you're likely to start feeling trimmer and have more energy. The diet she proposes is not exactly a hardship – berries and nuts over digestives, and nut butter over jam – but, unless you're creative, it could get expensive (see Chapter 9 for tips on keeping the cost down).

2. Watch your nutrient intake

If you're breastfeeding, be aware that a calorie deficit – eating fewer calories than you burn – could affect your milk supply. If you are weaning, and that is what you want, then it's your choice – but even if you're not breastfeeding, the body still needs extra nutrients for the repair work it has to do. This is why eating nutrient-rich food is so important right now – and why nutritionists recommend a prenatal/ postnatal vitamin to ensure you get what you and the baby need.

3. Trust your body
If you're craving a whole food, listen to your body and go for it. If your cravings are for junk food, there may be something in it – perhaps you need more salt, or carbohydrates, or you're eating too many carbohydrates and not enough protein to keep your blood sugar stable. Remember, however, that food manufacturers engineer foods to make them addictive. Use your instincts to decide whether your cravings are driven by a desire for nutrients or because something tastes wicked and delicious.

Can I diet whilst breastfeeding?
Probably – but everyone is different and evidence is limited. One study found that by restricting calorie intake to 1,500 a day, breastfeeding women did not significantly change the volume or composition of their milk. Another found low-carb diets like Atkins and the Paleo method are compatible with breastfeeding, as long as you eat enough fruit and vegetables to stay well nourished. Anecdotally, however, some women do find their milk supply drops when they reduce their food intake or increase their energy expenditure. A 1996 study found that breastfeeding women on a low-carb diet may experience fatigue, dehydration and energy loss. Dieticians recommend a supplement if you do try to lose weight whilst breastfeeding, and a 1999 study recommended that women eat a minimum of 100 grams a day of carbohydrates from wholegrain and cereals, fresh fruit and vegetables (equivalent to one jacket potato, a bowl of porridge and a banana).

20

Breasts

I've always found dark nipples more exotic than my own English-rose ones, and I hoped that mine would darken during pregnancy. It's a common side-effect – your skin makes more pigment, which gives you that stripe down the middle, the *linea nigra*. But my raspberry ripples stayed as pale and uninteresting as ever. The breasts on which they sit, however, became a constant source of fascination, going up and down and in and out like whoopee cushions.

During pregnancy, your boobs alone can increase in weight by almost a kilo. Mine felt colossal. I wore 32F nursing bras, but at times the fabric strained to contain them. The problem with having such enormous breasts was that no nice-looking bras were equipped to cope with them. I needed broad straps to stop them cutting into my shoulders, and an impossi-puzzle of clips at the back. These were not *brassières*, a word that conveys beauty and eroticism, but *Büstenhalter*, as they're called in German, which translates literally as breast holders. After some months, however, my breasts stabilised and, when I started weaning, became alarmingly insubstantial, prompting new concerns. Why had my once-firm tissue become rather pendulous and uninspiring? 'Like empty crisp packets,' as a friend bemoaned.

Pregnancy and the rollercoaster of breastfeeding don't

usually do your boobs any favours, and they don't go back to how they were before. While some women find theirs are bigger afterwards, many find they are smaller. Eight months in, I officially added 'breasts' to the list of things my darling boy had taken from me. When they weren't full of milk, which was most of the time, they offered no resistance to being pinched 'twixt finger and thumb; there was simply no density to them anymore. But, rather than put down this book and google breast-enhancement options, I suggest you take a minute to look kindly on your magic fun bags and think about all they have achieved.

Breasts are constantly changing and performing new miracles throughout a woman's life. Some of these acts of metamorphosis are, it must be said, less than desirable. In 2016, the *New Scientist* published an article entitled, 'Your boobs start to eat themselves after breastfeeding is over'. When you stop breastfeeding, it explained, the milk-producing cells you made when you were pregnant self-destruct, and then other cells come along and eat them. This 'massive cellular suicide', as the author colourfully described it, may help you to conceptualise why so many women end up with smaller boobs after pregnancy and breastfeeding than they had before. Delightful, isn't it? In addition, our ligaments often stretch, both during pregnancy and breastfeeding, which leaves the breasts sitting lower than before.

But another huge change is yet to come. Called involution, it refers to the replacement of glandular breast tissue with fat cells during the menopause; effectively the permanent closure of your milk factories. Part of the normal ageing process, involution has an upshot: it is believed to reduce your risk of breast cancer, as it's in the milk-producing glands where cancer originates.

Is there anything you can do about any of this? In terms of fighting these changes, not much, no. Breast-firming creams, exercise regimes and oestrogen-enhancing diets may claim to increase the density of breast tissue, but there isn't good evidence for these being effective. So, rather than spend money and energy that would be better directed elsewhere, it's healthier to make peace with your body, remember what it has achieved, and accept however your boobs look and feel now. After carrying around such weight in the early days of breastfeeding, I'm glad of my boobs' newfound lightness – and in awe of what they have done.

Breastfeeding aversion

Some women get the hang of breastfeeding only to find that their supply issues or sore nipples are replaced by another problem entirely – an alarming desire to run far away from their baby whenever it feeds, or to poke or pinch it to make it stop. Breastfeeding aversion can make you feel trapped and claustrophobic, 'touched out' and desperate for the baby to unlatch. It often affects women feeding their babies beyond six months, particularly when feeding on demand. Some women link it to their menstrual cycle, others find it has more to do with the mother–baby dynamic: exhaustion coupled with the desire for more independence, the pressure of other people's expectations, or problems with setting boundaries for yourself and your child. It's common to feel guilty about these thoughts, which is why Zainab Yate, a researcher and public health expert, established a website and wrote a book, *When Breastfeeding Sucks*, to provide women with resources and peer support. Yate published the first study into breastfeeding aversion in 2017,

after struggling to find any literature about the phenomenon when she suffered from it herself.

If you're experiencing something similar, make sure your
baby is suckling correctly, try to distract yourself during
feeds, try to get more sleep (being sleep-deprived is anecdotally linked to breastfeeding aversion), eat and drink well, and
take some time out if you can to restore a sense of personal
space. You can also consider whether it's linked to hormone
changes, for example the return of your periods.

> *Melissa had got over multiple bouts of mastitis and just
> started enjoying breastfeeding when she developed a
> sudden aversion to it:*
>
> 'It came completely out of the blue, like an emotional reac-
> tion to feeding – I suddenly felt touched out. I was in a happy
> place, and then all of a sudden I could not bear to feed, to
> have him on my skin, the whole process. And this feeling
> always peaked at bedtime when he'd feed for ages. It wasn't a
> rational thing, I just wanted to push him off me. No one talks
> about this and I think lots of women go through it. I remem-
> ber googling "breastfeeding aversion" because I thought this
> wasn't normal. The baby was sleeping well, I just couldn't
> bear to have him physically on top of me. My partner once
> came back and found me crying on the side of the bed, with
> the baby on the other side. It just wasn't rational, and it was
> really hard for my partner to understand that; I was happy,
> but I couldn't bring myself to feed him.'

Stopping breastfeeding

There is a huge amount of advice about establishing and
maintaining breastfeeding, but when you decide it's time to

stop, there's very little support out there. One friend, Meg, posted a request for advice in an online breastfeeding forum only to be reminded, unmercifully, 'this is a breastfeeding forum, we advise you don't stop.' Women are always encouraged to take up breastfeeding if they can, but then don't always find advice about ending it. I agonised for months over whether my son would ever go to sleep in the evenings without breastfeeding first. Everyone I asked told me it would be fine, he'd quickly adapt to having a cup of cow's milk instead. I didn't believe them. But it turns out they were absolutely right – it was really no issue at all.

For the nuts and bolts of stopping feeding, La Leche League offers invaluable advice. When it comes to you and your body, however, here's what you need to know.

You may have a come-down – When you start to cut out or stop breastfeeding, you might experience a come-down of sorts as your 'happy' hormones plummet once more. For some women, it happens when their babies start on solids and are feeding less, or when they cut out night feeds; for others, it's when they stop completely. It's not clear what exactly the relationship is between stopping breastfeeding and anxiety and depression – the research is thin, at best – but it is clear that a link exists. Levels of prolactin and oxytocin, happy hormones, drop when you stop, which can make you feel sad or grumpy. I have friends who needed anti-depressants when they stopped breastfeeding. Others noticed no difference at all. If you can, cutting it down slowly – over the course of weeks or even months – will help you adjust in body and mind.

Your boobs can become engorged again – If you don't or can't cut out breastfeeding over a long period of time (weeks, if not months), your boobs may be sore, painful and heavy with milk while they adapt. Engorgement can also lead to blocked ducts or mastitis (see Chapter 7). Express some milk if you need to, to reduce the discomfort.

You may feel unwell – The night sweats were probably at their worst a week or two after the baby was born, but they may come back when you stop breastfeeding. Women also report having headaches, feeling sick and experiencing mood swings.

Fertility returns – Some breastfeeding women find they start ovulating when their baby starts eating solids; for others, fertility doesn't return until a few months after they stop breastfeeding. According to the Lactational Amenorrhea Method of contraception, you could become pregnant once your baby is more than six months old, or as soon as it's not fully breastfed. And any decrease in milk production will make you more likely to start ovulating again, so consider contraception when you start weaning, even if you haven't yet had a period.

It can be stressful – For short periods, you may find your baby is crying and you can't – or don't want to – feed him or her, even though you know that doing so would provide relief for you both. This can make you feel horrible for the choices you've made. I technically weaned my son a number of times; having quit, we kept falling off the wagon because one or both of us needed it. In hindsight, it worked well; I didn't experience the symptoms associated with a sudden drop in hormones and, when we eventually stopped for good, neither of us really noticed. However you do it, remember that babies and young children are the most adaptable of all; you'll quickly find an alternative way of soothing them. Go gently and, if you can, be guided by their needs, and you may find it all goes very smoothly indeed.

My weaning story – and how I somehow made milk nine months later:
'*After a year of wearing nursing contraptions with ratchet straps, with weaning well underway, I decided to buy myself new bras. I chose a time when I could be alone and snuck into a department store. I tried on a delicate black bra with silver trim in my pre-pregnancy size. It fitted perfectly and, by some alchemy, I was transformed into an independent woman again. On my way out of the fitting rooms, I asked the kindly bra fitter to put the ratchet straps in the bin.*

'*My last few months of breastfeeding had been blissful. The milk came out slowly, and only when my son was suckling; no spillages, soaked shirts or stale milk smells. I was, finally, like the tranquil lady in my mum's picture. After cutting out feeds one by one, I eventually cut out the one I felt he was most addicted to – the bedtime feed. A sense of achievement and freedom washed over me; finally, I could go out in the evening while my husband put him to bed! After that, I fed him on an ad-hoc basis – whenever one of us needed it. And one day, at about 16 months, we just stopped – later than I'd expected, but not too late. Crucially, it felt right. My magic power left me, and my body was my own again.*

'*One crisp but sunny autumn day, nine months later, my son insisted on taking all his clothes off as we paddled, initially with wellies on, through a stream in a nearby wood. I tried to stop him, protesting about it being too cold, but he started to get cross with me. Remembering that he'd spent the first two years of his life watching me bathe in ice-cold water on a whim, I helped him to disrobe. He paddled naked for a while before we climbed the hill, aiming for a patch of sunlight. Sitting on the exposed roots of an ancient oak tree, I cradled his soft, naked body as we basked in the warm rays. A familiar feeling of warmth filled my chest and, when I looked down at him, whooomp, there it was again, the let-down.*

'Curious, I extracted a bit of what had come out using the end of my finger, just to be sure. Before I could inspect it, with the reflexes of a snake, my toddler darted his head forward and licked it, then grinned at me. I'm not sure which of us was more surprised by this sequence of events; we both lay back, helpless with giggles. Breasts are wondrous, if not peculiar, things.'

21

Skin, Hair and Nails

Had it been the hair on my legs falling out after giving birth, it would have been welcome. Instead, it was the hair on my head. Along with brittle nails and spotty skin, here are some of the irksome cosmetic issues that can occur after birth.

Skin

Just like during puberty, the hormonal and physical changes in your body mean you may be more prone to skin disorders like acne and dry skin. This extends to your intimate areas, too. Pelvic health physiotherapists recommend using a vaginal moisturiser after birth to restore the skin's condition.

Stretch marks – The skin of your belly and boobs will have been stretched by your extra size and weight, so stretch marks might be another vestige of your pregnancy. If you didn't apply your body oil when you were pregnant, don't worry about it – there is no reason to believe that any of the products marketed as preventing stretch marks actually work. They moisturise the skin, which can help with other side-effects, such as itching and dryness, but do nothing for the collagen beneath the surface, which is responsible for the formation of stretch marks. Nor should you worry too much about moisturising them now – studies show that neither almond oil, cocoa butter, olive oil or vitamin E help the marks to fade. Just two substances have been shown to make stretch marks less noticeable: hyaluronic acid, a sugar found naturally in our skin, and tretinoin, a vitamin-A derivative that is typically used to treat acne, both of which are available on prescription or from specialist skincare companies.

Eczema/dry skin – A lot of women experience dry skin for a while after pregnancy. Keep moisturising, ideally with an unperfumed cream or natural oil (dermatologists recommend sunflower oil as it's safe, inexpensive and widely available) and if it's eczema, don't worry – it's likely to pass. Moisturise, and if it doesn't get better, see your doctor. Short-term use of topical steroids like hydrocortisone cream is considered safe while breastfeeding, if your doctor recommends it.

Melasma – Known as a 'pregnancy mask' or chloasma, this refers to the brown or greyish pigmentation that can appear on the face during pregnancy and affects as many as 50 per cent of us. Melasma has no physical symptoms and is usually more noticeable in the summer than in the winter. There is currently no cure, but treatments can help the marks to fade – although it's a good idea to wait a few months after the birth as they may go away on their own. The British Association of Dermatologists suggests avoiding known triggers, including UV light (keep out of the sun or wear SPF 30+ suncream), contraceptive pills and hormone replacement therapy. Hydroquinone cream, which stops cells producing melanin, is commonly prescribed, but it's not without risks – it can irritate the skin, in rare cases can make the problem worse, and can only be used for a few weeks at a time. Retinoid creams and certain acids like azelaic acid can help, but they can also irritate the skin. A dermatologist may be able to recommend a retinoid cream that also contains a topical steroid, to prevent the irritation.

Acne – While you recover from the hormonal tornado that took you back to adolescence, you may feel a bit teenagerish in the skin department. Plenty of topical treatments are safe if you're breastfeeding, both over the counter and on prescription. Benzoyl peroxide is widely available and generally considered safe, but it can irritate and dry out skin. Products containing azelaic acid, salicylic acid, glycolic acid or sulphur can be effective but less harsh on the skin.

It's recommended that you avoid topical retinoid treatments like retinol during early pregnancy – retinoids are vitamin-A derivatives, which work on acne and fine lines – on the basis that taking the acne medication isotretinoin (known as Accutane or Roaccutane), a retinoid taken orally, *is* known to cause birth defects (even though retinoids are not well absorbed by the skin and no studies have shown a link between topical retinoids and birth defects). The absence of research into the interaction between breastmilk and retinoids means that many dermatologists urge you to be safe and avoid them while you're breastfeeding as well – although it's considered highly unlikely that doing so will have any ill-effects; the reason it's not recommended during pregnancy is because excessive vitamin A intake can interfere with foetal development in early pregnancy, and you're well past that stage by now.

Hair

The time I spent in communal showers during my adolescence left me with an aversion to stray hair stuck to tiles or clogging up plugholes. During pregnancy, my thick, curly hair grew long and luscious; it barely fell out at all. It was only about two months afterwards that the problems started. I was never concerned about losing too much – I had a lot to start with – but I was horrified by the way it seemed to come out in clumps for months on end.

What happened next was less unpleasant but more conspicuous. Around seven months after the baby was born, short tufts of hair started to grow upwards, with a counter-gravitational frizz that had me looking like a mushroom cloud. When I tried to hide it with a high ponytail, I was left with a band of short hair underneath that stuck to my forehead and temples like a monk's cap. I was growing a second layer of hair, like a snake grows a second skin.

When you're not pregnant, around 85 to 90 per cent of the hairs on your head are growing at any one time. The remaining 10 per cent are resting, before they fall out to make way for new hair. The cycle of replacement, from new growth to falling out, normally takes two to four years. The abrupt hormonal changes that come with pregnancy and childbirth, however, can cause up to 30 per cent of your hair to stop growing and enter the resting phase, which lasts around three months, before they all start falling out. Little is known about *telogen effluvium*, as this is called, but it is thought to affect over half of all new mums and requires no treatment, just patience and regular cleaning of your shower drain. Your hair might feel thin for a while, but it should fall out evenly so you shouldn't see any balding patches. If you do notice patchy areas and are concerned, make an appointment with your doctor. Eventually, in order to cope with this short, immature hair that refused to obey the rules of the flock, I booked an appointment with a trendier-than-normal hairdresser and started afresh with a short crop.

Weak nails

Charlotte Pearson, Mummy Fever blogger:
'Every single one of my fingernails had snapped off within 24 hours of my daughter's birth. It was totally bizarre.'

A lot of women complain of weak, brittle or ridged nails during and after pregnancy. It barely needs saying that hormones are to blame. Nails typically grow faster than usual during pregnancy; for some women, nail strength and appearance improve, others see them get worse. American obstetrician and gynaecologist Amos Grünebaum, who founded the website babyMed, says that the first enemy of weak nails is water. Wear gloves for washing-up or cleaning, and moisturise to repair the nails as you would dry skin. It can take three to six months for your fingernails to go back to normal, he says – and nine months for your toenails to do the same!

22

Sex, Intimacy and Fertility

The sex. When does it go back to normal? I asked a few people this question and didn't get many encouraging answers. Some glazed over, leaving my question to hang in the air. Others groaned and then moved on to a less-uncomfortable subject. A few cracked jokes about how making another baby was going to be a stretch. Only two surprised me with their honesty. One launched into an explanation of her problem, which was this: ever since their first baby, her partner had refused to go near her nipples, which were her favourite erogenous zone. Their baby was now two, she'd stopped breastfeeding months ago, and was doing everything she could to get her partner 'back on the boob' – but he still wasn't going for it. In stark contrast, the other looked me in the eye and said, 'I'd be perfectly happy if I never saw a penis again.'

As with a lot of female-only health complaints, the research into postpartum sex is limited; the number of studies on male sexual dysfunction far outweighs those on female sexual dysfunction, even though it is more common in women than in men. (While you can get Viagra in the post, next-day delivery, there is no comparable option for us.)

On average, couples have sex for the first time eight to ten weeks after birth. While some women have no problems at all, it's common to experience some sort of pain for the first 12 months; a quarter of women who had no significant tearing will find sex painful for that year, over a third of those who had a second-degree tear, and just over half of those who had an OASI, according to a recent study of over 500 women in Denmark.

The fact that doctors, nurses and midwives often don't have the necessary skills to help with intimacy issues can make it seem like our sex lives aren't important. But any problems need to be talked about and taken seriously, because negative experiences can lead to a vicious circle of fear and failure and can have an impact on mental health.

Some women worry that their partners aren't, and won't ever again be, interested in sex with them, because of what they saw during the birth or how they now look. Others wish their partners *weren't* interested, either because sex is painful or traumatic, or because they get more than enough groping from their baby. Many women mistakenly think their partner wants sex, whereas all they really want is intimacy. It can feel daunting to broach subjects like this, particularly if you haven't had to discuss such sensitive issues in any depth before – as a lot of us haven't. And it can take a while to understand that it's not the sex, but the intimacy and communication that really counts, so remember to talk to and trust your partner.

On my son's first day of nursery, my friend Wendy said I should do something for myself. Wendy never usually paints her nails but, after she dropped her daughter off, she came home, sat on her terrace overlooking our beautiful valley, and painted her fingernails. My toenails desperately needed painting, and this book also needed writing; I was itching to get started. But there was one thing more pressing than getting back to work, and it was doing something for me and Philip, as a couple, alone, with no fear of interruption.

We dropped him off at nursery together, came home and melted into each other's arms for the first time in weeks. 'We're still together,' I said afterwards, failing to hide my relief that the emotional and physical bonds we'd forged as a couple felt as strong as ever.

When to have sex?

There is no answer to this question, but common suggestions are when you feel ready, when you stop bleeding, and when you've been checked and signed off by a doctor (not, like me, when curiosity gets the better of you). Prepare your partner for the fact that it might be a long and, at times, bumpy road back to regular sex – and by that I mean sex when you actually *want* to prioritise sex over sleep, sex that doesn't involve the odd stabbing pain, sex that isn't punctuated by embarrassing noises or squawks of discomfort, and sex that doesn't leave you covered in milk or have you imagining your husband as your baby. (Get him to read Parts 1 and 4 of this book if you want him to understand what you may be going through.)

Whatever feels right for you, make sure you communicate it. Often, women who aren't ready to have penetrative sex find themselves avoiding any physical intimacy – either because they are scared of what it will lead to, or because they don't want to give their partner false expectations. This can make the partner feel rejected or leave them thinking that all intimacy has gone from their relationship. Sex can become the elephant in the room, partners can start to lose confidence in themselves, and it becomes a cycle of avoidance and denial that affects both you and your relationship.

Good communication is the key to avoiding this, and there's plenty of fun to be had without a penis entering your vagina.

The tradition of abstinence

In sub-Saharan Africa, the traditional period of abstinence after childbirth is anything from three months to over a year, often until the baby can walk or is weaned. If it's broken, people believe that certain illnesses may befall mother and child. This makes sense given that contraception can be scarce in Africa, polygamy is common, and it's universally recommended that women wait at least 18 months before becoming pregnant again for the sake of their bodies. As access to contraception improves, modern healthcare supplants traditional medicine, and long-established practices give way to modern thinking, the period of abstinence is declining rapidly. Back in 1990, couples in Tanzania waited on average six and a half months; in 2010, they waited a little under three months. Now, the average wait in East Africa seems to be more in line with Europe, just six to eight weeks.

Ménage à moi

While we crack jokes about male masturbation and assume fondly that most menfolk are at it, even in the post-*Sex and the City* era we are still not that comfortable about women doing the same. But we should be, because if you're postpartum and thinking about sex again, experts say that masturbating is often the best place to start. You're in control of how far you go, it's exploratory, and it can be inclusive and fun if you do it together. The wonderful women at Liverpool Women's Hospital's physiotherapy department want to make a *ménage à moi* as acceptable for women as it is for men. It doesn't necessarily mean you are ready to have sex again, they say – it can be a stepping-stone, and one that stops intimacy from becoming a hurdle that you have to get over. Plus, some men get too anxious to enjoy sex during pregnancy or postpartum – they can worry about hurting the baby, hurting you, or not helping your healing. It can be easier, particularly when things feel different, to explore yourself, with or without your partner involved. Just don't expect too much – your orgasms may well be underwhelming to start with.

What to expect

Whether you had a vaginal birth or a caesarean, sex may feel a bit different to start with. It can help to have an idea of what to expect; while persistent issues are common, in most cases women find that things settle down fairly quickly.

Faint + feeble – The first time you try penetrative sex, you may find it rather like 'waving a flag in a warehouse', as one physiotherapist told me. And that's not because it's gaping, she added, in response to my squawk of recognition, but because of the numbness – which apparently can last for months after birth. As she spoke, memories of our first postpartum sexual escapade came flooding back. No one told us not to have sex until six weeks, as the NHS recommends, so we tried it rather sooner – not because I felt sexy, but because I'm innately curious and wanted to know if things still worked. And they did, albeit rather like she described.

Your orgasms are also likely to a bit feeble for a while; a landmark study back in the 1970s confirmed that women's sex organs simply don't climax as vigorously as they used to for a few months after birth. Don't worry – this should only be temporary; they should come back soon enough. Mind-blowing orgasms, or the absence thereof, are another reason to do your pelvic floor exercises; orgasms are bigger and stronger when these muscles are in fine fettle.

Discomfort – A lot of women find sex uncomfortable to start with. As the Irish author Anne Enright wrote in her memoir, *Making Babies*: 'Welcome to the big secret: it hurts.' Beyond the first few times, however, experts say that you shouldn't put up with pain but get a pelvic health physiotherapist to take a look; painful sex at the start is common, but it should go away.

Take it slowly and be patient and kind to yourself. And get some lube (see page 312). You may find that one position is better than another, because of the location of your cervix or sensitive tissue, for example. Talk about it and navigate it together – or go back to 'outercourse', as it's called, which is basically anything other than penetrative sex. (For more on pain, see page 314).

Still healing – Scar tissue can cause problems, so therapists and physios recommend you look carefully at what's happening to your wound while it's healing and, when the time is right, gently probe the tissue to see if there's any pain or discomfort. Ask your partner to feel around and say when it hurts. Light massage brings circulation to the area, which promotes healing. When you do have sex, use what you've learned to make it feel good.

Libido – It is considered 'normal', whatever that means, to lose all libido for the first six or seven weeks after giving birth. Having sex can seem like an audacious waste of

energy and time. You may have injuries and physical trauma
to grapple with, psychological issues, huge changes to your
body and its functions, a weak pelvic floor, engorged or leaky
breasts – if you're breastfeeding, your body has become your
baby's by now – or just feel exhausted, stressed and sleep-
deprived. These are simply not things that leave a woman
feeling horny, so try not to worry about it.

A reduced sex drive becomes abnormal, according to a
recent review of all studies, when your libido is persistently
reduced or absent, causing distress in your relationship. The
root cause is usually one of two things: you're either experiencing painful or difficult sex, or you're preoccupied with
the baby or your own post-natal complications. Pain is the
more common one (see page 314).

Dryness – Pelvic health physios bemoan the fact that dryness,
an almost universal problem in postnatal women, can be so
taboo. They proudly tote tubes of lube in their handbags,
and recommend clients use a vaginal moisturiser as well to
combat the effects of oestrogen depletion, which can make
you even more tender down there. It's very normal to have
less of your body's natural lubrication for six months or
more after birth because of low oestrogen levels, especially if
you're breastfeeding. The dryness can cause pain or embarrassment, and that in turn can further impact your desire for
sex. The best way around this is to use a lubricant from the
start, and to moisturise with either a dedicated product or
coconut oil. If you don't use some form of lubrication, you're
setting yourself up for discomfort.

Visual changes – If you had a vaginal birth, it takes a while
to get your head around the fact that your vagina is probably

not going to go back to exactly how it was before. 'Frilly' was one word used by a pelvic physio that appealed to me – it sounds far nicer than 'flappy', which is how a male gynaecologist, referred to in the section on prolapses, once described a friend's. With time, things do firm up and settle down, but as the American sex therapist Kathe Wallace said, 'confidence is knowing the truth', and accepting that you may not look or feel exactly the same again.

> *Alex, who had her last child nearly a decade ago, remembers feeling crestfallen at her broken body, but she is fitter than ever today:*
> *'I remember sex after both of my children really being not that good. It's just not – a baby's gone through there! I remember thinking, oh shit, is this it now? Is that what it's going to feel like forever more? No one has these conversations. Your boobs are leaking, your gut's wobbling around – oh for God's sake, I thought. But, nearly ten years after my last birth, my body has never been in better shape. I have never been stronger, healthier, firmer – I've never been more proud of it. And it's important to talk about these things as well, as a way of reassuring and inspiring other women.'*

Does how you gave birth have a bearing on postpartum sex?

Episiotomies in particular are a risk factor for problems (more so than spontaneous tears), but beyond that the jury is out on whether perineal trauma is to blame for women's tanking sexual proclivity after birth. In one camp are the scientists who blame vaginal births for the difficulties women have with postnatal sex, and in the other camp are the scientists who think that the mode of delivery – whether you had a C-section or vaginal birth – has little bearing on your ability to get back in the sack. As a 2010 review of the research says, this difference of opinion makes it very difficult to advise women who want a caesarean because of fears that a vaginal birth will destroy their sex lives.

Where in the world would a woman base her birth plan on what's best for her sex life, I wondered? Well, I'll give you a clue: it's one of the world's largest swimwear exporters, and it has a bikini wax named after it.

Brazil, the capital of carnival and plastic surgery, is also the capital of caesareans, reportedly because Brazilian women do indeed worry about the impact that a vaginal birth will have on their sex lives. Elective caesareans started out as a status symbol but became pandemic; 55 per cent of births are now via caesarean. But doctors and scientists caution that Brazilian women are misguided if they're choosing caesareans to safeguard sex: contrary to what you might expect, painful sex is also common after caesareans. According to a number of studies, the chances of having painful or problematic sex after a caesarean versus a vaginal birth are roughly equal. According to a recent British study, any sort of intervention (elective caesarean included) carries double the risk of painful or problematic sex at 18 months postpartum compared to a spontaneous labour with no significant tearing. The cause of pain can be muscular, or can relate to scarring, because even though the baby didn't come out of your vagina, it still came from the opposite end of the same tube, which underwent major changes.

When problems persist

I didn't realise that 'touched out' was a common refrain until I experienced it myself – when the physical demands of a newborn leads to a loss of physical autonomy, to the point that your body can no longer feel like your own. I would frequently explain to Philip how the baby's tiny hands and mouth had claimed every inch of my body, leaving nothing for anyone else. The physical intimacy you have with your child can be heartstoppingly beautiful, but also overwhelming and claustrophobic at times. With hindsight, the time I spent breastfeeding was very short-lived, and I'm so grateful for the intimacy we shared. Now, almost three years on, it feels like I'm the one constantly demanding cuddles and my baby is the one who gets touched out.

If feeling touched out is affecting you and your partner's relationship, a sex therapist recommended reframing intimacy for a while so that it's purely about you. Make your partner understand that you need the sort of touch and engagement that doesn't feel demanding, for example, by building intimacy in non-sexual ways. Ask him to give you a head or foot massage, take a bath together, or hold each other until you feel your shoulders drop as the tension falls away. I find a game of Scrabble can rebuild intimacy and connection in a way that watching television can't. Just try to avoid sex becoming one more thing on your burgeoning to-do list; instead, try to see your (limited) adult time as an opportunity to lose yourself and find some pleasure outside of the mundane.

In her motherhood memoir, *My Wild and Sleepless Nights*, the British author Clover Stroud likens sex to being on strong drugs, and describes it as the place where she goes to escape motherhood and all of its associated demands. Sex enables her to shut out her children, literally and metaphorically, and to be herself again. 'I can't really do anything about the kids when my wrists are pinned to the bed,' she writes. It's rare to see a mother of small children describing sex with such unbounded enthusiasm, but I found her take on it – sex as a celebration of privacy, intimacy and adulthood – compelling. I often struggled with the *idea* of sex – I would feel physically drained by the baby pawing and sucking at my body. Yet once we were between the sheets, everything would slip away and I'd lose myself in the pleasure of it. Thanks to Stroud, I was able to reframe it: it stopped being another demand on my body, and started being a way to escape those demands.

Breastfeeding and sex

A 2016 study found that over twice as many breastfeeding women had problems with sex at six months, compared to non-breastfeeding women. This didn't surprise me; when I was breastfeeding, my body had a higher calling and my boobs had an aversion to anything other than (and sometimes including) my baby's touch. A more recent study also associated breastfeeding with being dissatisfied about your body; again, this doesn't surprise me, because it's hard to feel sexy when your breasts could, at any moment, shower your partner in milk.

Laxity

If, after about twelve weeks, you feel little during sex, it may be that you have some laxity in your vagina that needs correcting with pelvic floor muscle training. It's common to be more lax if you've had more than one child, if your baby was large, or if you had an instrumental birth. See Strength training in Chapter 15, and consider an assessment with a pelvic health physio.

Fanny farts

If you find you make more noises during sex than you used to (and I'm not talking about moans of pleasure), you are not alone. Having a percussive vagina (often called queefing, a word that has yet to make it into the *Oxford English Dictionary*) is one of the few things to make urinary incontinence seem like dinner-table talk.

The fact that you queef – during sex or perhaps yoga – is not information that you're likely to volunteer, which means we often don't realise how common it is. If you do get any wind in your vagina, you have no warning or control over when and how it comes out, which is why it can be so perturbing. During a yoga class, when queefs are common, a lone parp will make you stare intently at your mat, praying there are no more to come. During sex, a barrage of queefs might induce helpless giggles – or leave you mortified.

There are a few common reasons for fanny farting: because something – for instance, a penis – pushes air in there; weak pelvic floor muscles allow air in when the pressure in your abdomen drops; or, according to biomechanics expert Katy Bowman, weak core muscles that, whenever your hips go above your ribcage, allow your organs to create a vacuum that sucks the air in like a syringe. Rarely, queefs can be signs of something serious, like a fistula (which is any abnormal hole between the vagina and one of the adjacent organs such as the bladder or bowels). But it's usually just weak muscles plus yoga or a penis that are to blame. Jane

Simpson, London's pelvic guru and author of *The Pelvic Floor Bible*, emphasises that it's not something you should put up with. Work on strengthening your core muscles, including the pelvic floor, or see a pelvic health physiotherapist who can assess you and show you what you need to do.

Ongoing problems with sex

Treating stubborn issues – from low libido to persistent pain – can be immensely complex due to the interplay between mental and physical wellbeing, and the deeply personal nature of it all. Good women's health physiotherapists should recognise this and be well attuned to a woman's need for discretion and sensitivity; they are trained to recognise and manage symptoms of mental trauma as well as its more obvious physical counterparts. There are also psychotherapists who specialise in sex and relationship therapy.

> *Emma Mathews, psychotherapist and former midwife specialising in perinatal mental health, explains how she goes about treating clients postpartum:*
> *'Sex isn't just a physical thing; we're talking about emotional processes as well. In terms of motivation for a woman to be sexual, there has to be emotional intimacy – the relationship has got to be OK, and the woman has got to feel OK with herself. Often, women can be sexually neutral in terms of drive; whilst not totally averse to the idea of sex, they wouldn't particularly feel the desire to initiate it. I see lots of heterosexual couples and they are quite distressed because the guy's libido is a lot higher than the woman's, and it's always the man that initiates sex. This is only a problem if the woman can't become motivated or aroused when she's*

presented with some sexual stimuli. There are times, often around ovulation, that a woman may be more inclined to initiate sex as the biological drive is there. When the woman is sexually neutral and the right buttons are pressed, then she can become sexually aroused. If the arousal increases, they'll carry on. And if there's emotional and physical satisfaction, it'll feed back into the next time – because even though she didn't have the initial desire, it turned out to be pretty good.

'If a woman has had difficulties, if sex has been painful or if there have been emotional difficulties, then once she gets that stimulus, she is likely to have negative thoughts and beliefs, and then what we call catastrophic misinterpretations – for example, I'll be in agony, I'll be out of control, I'll lose control of my bowels, I'll be embarrassed or I'm not normal. Those thoughts lead to a negative emotional response, which can be fear, anger or shame; when people experience these kinds of emotions, their vaginal muscles can contract or they can notice pain more intensely. They can put in place various behaviours to try to keep themselves safe, for example, avoiding or trying to control any genital contact. Life then becomes limited by attempts to avoid and control sexual contact, which leads to them feeling stuck, anxious and depressed.

'A proportion of women will have developed this due to their traumatic experience of childbirth – and it's not always the actual birth; it can be problems that happen afterwards, such as everything that goes along with having a third- or fourth-degree tear and how it affects you emotionally. Sensations can bring back memories of the trauma – we're talking about PTSD symptoms. So if there is psychological trauma, I make sure they have an assessment and treatment for that. If you have PTSD, you feel a constant sense of threat and *need to protect yourself. Women develop coping strategies as a result, and unhelpful beliefs about the birth itself, where they blame others or themselves, or about the world and their future.*

'In psychosexual therapy, I firstly initiate a sex ban, because when a sexual problem develops, the person who has developed it often interprets any physical touch as something that may lead to sexual contact, so they avoid all forms of intimacy with their partner. This can keep the problem going and cause wider relationship problems. At least with a sex ban in place they can be intimate and touch each other in a nonsexual and mindful way without fear of where the physical touch may lead. I would usually give some solo tasks for the woman to do in terms of vaginal dilators or vibrators. I also give partner tasks. They can add in more focus on genital touch, but it very much depends on the client's goals. If the sexual problem has developed as a result of a third- or fourth-degree tear, I'd want to work in conjunction with a physio who can check out the physical side of the problem, whilst I work on the psychological side.

'It's important to remember that sex doesn't particularly need to be penetrative sex; so many people have this idea that unless it involves a penis in an orifice then it's not proper sex. That's not true and as long as you enjoy it and it's consensual, it's OK.'

Rewinding sex

Sexual contact runs the full gamut, from cuddling and kissing to things I can't imagine any new mother wanting (unless she was lucky enough never to discover haemorrhoids). Your postnatal experience will greatly determine where you fall on this spectrum – but if your sex drive doesn't recover, rewinding things can help. Thanks to two American academics who pioneered sex research in the first half of the last century, Masters and Johnson (known as the 'masters of sex'), this is an easy way of getting out of sex ruts. Sensate focus, as it's known, works by hitting the 'reset' button on a stalemate. Firstly, neither of you should make any attempt to have sex. This works on the basis that fear is getting in the way of good sex, and you can get rid of it by removing all expectations and rewinding your intimacy to where it began. Once you're both relaxed, spend a night doing just one thing: kissing. Do it as enthusiastically as you like, but do no more than you would have done at a well-lit teenage disco. Next, spend a night going one step further – touching bodies, but not breasts or bits. By now, you may feel more enthusiastic about the prospect of sex than you did at the start. The next level involves hands and genitals, so you can orgasm (although it's not the goal), but again – no penetrative sex. Next, you can finally have penetrative sex – but it mustn't go on for long and there can be no orgasm! Repeat that on a few evenings until you graduate to the final level, when you can at last have normal sex – and it should by now be without any of the anxieties or complexities you felt before. (But, if they do creep in, I'm afraid it's back to level one again.)

Periods and fertility

Everyone is different, but if you're not breastfeeding, your period may start somewhere between three and eight weeks after you give birth. Most women don't ovulate on their first cycle but, by the second cycle, things should be getting back to normal (although your periods may be heavier, longer and more painful than before, in part because your uterus is likely a little bigger). The NHS warns that if you have blood clots in a period for a week or more, or have much heavier bleeding than before, you should speak to a health professional. If you breastfeed, you might not have your first period again until you drop the night feeds, start weaning, or stop feeding altogether. Your first period might be heavier than before, contain clots, and be more (or less painful) than before. You may also have worse PMS.

If you're breastfeeding and you haven't had a period, you could still be fertile because you may – unbeknown to you – just have ovulated and be about to have a period; we all know someone who got caught out by this (see LAM, on page 323). If you don't breastfeed, it's possible to get pregnant as little as three weeks after you've given birth. Once you've had a period, it can take another six months for your body to re-establish a regular menstrual rhythm. And, if you're breastfeeding but having regular periods, you may find you can't conceive because the breastfeeding hormones thin the lining of the womb, which prevents a fertilised egg from implanting.

Contraception

The NHS website says that a family planning adviser should discuss contraception with you before you leave the hospital. Thankfully, no such advice made it to me; I dread to think what I would have said to someone asking about my plans for contraception while I was still in the throes of birth. If you are thinking about it immediately, however, condoms, an implant, injection or the progesterone-only pill can all be used straight afterwards. A coil can usually be fitted four weeks after giving birth (but it's also possible to insert one within 48 hours of birth).

I had a copper coil before getting pregnant and it worked so well I never thought about it. After my baby, when my periods eventually came back, however, I had another copper coil fitted and it was ghastly. For the first time, I had heavy, painful periods and bi-monthly cramping. After birth, it's possible that the surface area of your uterus will be double what it was – which is why many women complain of heavier periods after childbirth (and perhaps why I had a different relationship with the copper coil).

You can expect another conversation about contraception at your six-week check. For many, it's still an academic discussion at that point – either because you have no interest in sex, or because you're breastfeeding (see Lactational Amenorrhea Method, below). Still, all options will be available, and you should take them seriously if you don't think you'd cope with two under two.

Lactational Amenorrhea Method (LAM)

If you're breastfeeding your baby on demand, it's less than six months old, and you feed it at least every four hours during the day and six hours at night, you are covered by LAM, which is 98 per cent successful at preventing pregnancy – a similar failure rate to other forms of contraception. Because it's difficult to be sure you're maintaining this, health professionals advise you to use another form of contraception to be absolutely certain – especially after the first few months.

23

Psychological Transitions

Postnatal anxiety and depression can come tumbling down on you at any time in the first year or so. For me, the most challenging time was not the first few weeks or even months but about four months in. Tiredness accumulates and, just as we were recovering from the first three months and starting to feel confident of a good night's sleep, our apparently good sleeper started waking up at night. We didn't know what to do, and early parenthood felt not like a challenge but a torturous joke devised specifically for us by a malevolent god. It felt far harder than the first few months and, without the support of friends and family, I may have become depressed.

Almost half of mums with postnatal depression cite loneliness as a key trigger. Research shows, however, that only half of those who suffer ever get formal help. The number one cure, according to a survey by the NCT, is not drugs or therapy but simply having a peer group – other mums to talk to. Psychologists, midwives and health visitors agree: if you can find someone to share things with, you'll be a happier and more confident mother.

I never mastered the art of making friends through babies, however. For me, making real friends has usually involved misbehaviour, which forges the bonds of mutual insubordination: climbing something forbidden, an impromptu wild night out, or leaping into a lake in our underwear. It's hard to break rules or do anything spontaneous when you have a small baby, so I felt rather uninspired – and uninspiring – when it came to making new friends.

I discovered, however, that you don't need many friends to support you – just one or two will do. My closest local friend got me through countless afternoons when the hours of boredom and loneliness stretched ahead like a tightrope over a gorge. And then there was my mum, who would drive for half an hour just to sit with the baby while I sat in the same room and worked.

Everyone would tell me that the baby stage 'goes so quickly', I should make the most of it before it's gone. In her motherhood memoir, Clover Stroud clings onto her newborn with such force it's almost like she really does want it to remain an infant. It's true, it does go like a flash when you look back. But it doesn't always feel that way when you're in it. I would look with envy at mothers whose toddlers said rude words and ran away. There's no doubt that I was growing to love our son with a force that I didn't think possible, but I often had my sights on the milestones and the finish line, when the baby would become a little boy. For that reason, I hope I'll never preach to a struggling new mum about how quickly the time goes, because looking back warps your perspective. It feels like time moves faster now that we have a child – and, as I write, we'll soon start again with the second – but when you're in the thick of it with a tiny baby on your own, an hour can be an eternity.

Imogen spent the first three months of her daughter's life with her husband around – but then they moved to another country and he started work. After a doula advised she sleep-train her baby, things started to fall apart:

'My husband would go off every day and I'd feel all alone. I turned to reading all sorts of books, especially about sleep. When the baby was three months, a virtual doula recommended we start this draconian sleep-training schedule. For two weeks, she would cry for 30 or 40 minutes before she'd go to sleep. She'd rock her head back and forth. "She's finding her sleep position," the doula would say! No, she's writhing in agony, I was thinking. But I felt that sleep-training was what I needed to do to be a good mum.

'After the first night, she stopped looking me in the eye, as if she wanted to punish me. It was the most scary thing I've ever dealt with. Was I doing her damage? Was our relationship ever going to be the same? For three months we'd been in sync and that had gone. We moved her out of our bedroom and I spent hours staring at the video monitor, thinking, does she need me? It all felt a lot more dramatic because I didn't have anybody to talk me down. When she was crying, I would scream at my husband because I felt her crying so keenly.

'After two weeks, she started sleeping through the night. But I suddenly found her really fussy when she was feeding and she would come on and off the breast. I didn't know what that meant; I never thought she might not be getting milk. When we saw a paediatrician for something else, he said, "My goodness, she's not gained weight for a month. You obviously need to start formula, it's not working with breastfeeding."

'Potentially giving up breastfeeding represented losing my "amazing mother" status and admitting it was all a mess; it felt like the most important failure I'd ever had. I did try *formula but she didn't even take a bottle. The days would turn into yawning stretches of time where I would feel like I needed to feed her constantly and, if she didn't want it, I would feel personally rejected, like a terrible mother. Then I would start crying and she would start crying; we spent days in a soup of stress and tears. Every morning my husband would leave and I would almost be begging him not to go. It felt like the worst thing to be facing a day with her on my own.*

'I started waking her every three hours at night to feed, to get my supply up, so I wasn't getting more than a two-hour stretch of sleep. That's when I really lost my shit and went into postnatal anxiety. It was so acute, I lost touch with reality in a way I've never done before. I thought the baby was starving and looked emaciated when actually she looked fine. I couldn't look at her without thinking it's all my fault. I became obsessed with my let-down; I thought I couldn't feel it and that she wasn't getting any milk. And then I'd be trying to control my thinking to bring on the let-down, thinking about waves of milk, telling myself she will live, and then thinking about not thinking about the let-down; it was insane. I think I was making it up actually – I was letting-down fine, but thinking I wasn't was a way to blame myself.

'This lasted about two months and there were times when I was a little bit suicidal. I used to tell my husband that I was going to jump off the balcony. I was not well. It's weird to think of yourself out of your mind with anxiety, especially as I hadn't had mental health problems before. The thing that got me out of it was moving back to the US, where I'm from. It was on the plane ride back that she started feeding happily again – maybe she sensed my relief. She was six months by then and it was like coming out of water. Was this all in my

*head, I wondered? I think so. The relief continued to come
in waves. When I saw a breastfeeding consultant in the US,
she said, you know, it might not have been you, it might have
been your baby. I remember sobbing hearing that, it was such
a revelation – that I hadn't necessarily caused all of this. I
had made mistakes but it was a two-way relationship; we'd
gotten through it together and it wasn't all my fault. From
then on, breastfeeding was the beautiful bonding thing that
it is for some people throughout.'*

Matrescence

If you read Chapter 1 on the making of a mother, you'll
remember the word matrescence. Dana Raphael, an American scientist and founder of the doula movement, coined the
term back in the 1970s when the natural birth movement was
gathering strength and Ina May Gaskin was pioneering her
empowering, earth-mother version of childbirth. Anthropologists and psychologists now use the word to describe the
birth of a mother and transition to motherhood.

My understanding of what this transition means has
deepened over the past three years as I have come to understand myself better, and heard other women talk about their
own journeys – each unique but united by a rapid learning curve and ever-deepening insight. Just as a baby spends
months developing in utero before being born, as the psychiatrist Daniel Stern writes in his book, *The Birth of a Mother*,
a mother needs months to develop psychologically – and the
birth of her new identity can be as rewarding but also as
arduous as that of her child.

Dr Alexandra Sacks is a psychiatrist who hosts a podcast
series called Motherhood Sessions about the mother's

experience. Writing in the *New York Times*, she describes how having insight into our emotions can make us more in control of our behaviour; knowing about the challenges that new mothers commonly face can normalise and validate how we are feeling, and help us to cope with them.

So what exactly are the challenges that women commonly encounter as they become mothers? Firstly, Sacks says, your family dynamics change. In creating a baby you have created a family. Your baby is very small and lacks the faculty of speech, but they will make crucial changes to you and your partner's relationship, as well as your relationship with your parents, siblings, and even friends. Indeed, I found that having a baby changes your relationship with everything; its irresistibly sweet wrecking ball knows no bounds. After ours was born, I spent over a year renegotiating the terms of our new love triangle, trying to soften the edges and bring the three of us together into something that looked more like a circle. It took some work to get there, but Philip and I ended up closer than before. On the other hand, our son's birth had a positive effect on my relationship with my parents from the start.

The second challenge that you need to get used to, according to Sacks, is ambivalence – having mixed or contradictory feelings about something or someone. It is what Rachel Cusk describes so well in her memoir of motherhood, *A Life's Work*: 'Birth is not merely that which divides women from men: it also divides women from themselves.' It changes our understanding of everything, including our very existence; once someone else has existed inside you, Cusk writes, they continue to exist within your sphere of consciousness even after their birth, so that you are no longer yourself when you are with them, and you are no longer yourself when you are without them. Leaving them can thus feel as difficult as staying with them.

I fought a constant urge to be without my baby in order to be myself again, and yet I felt compelled by the need to press his little body against mine and to shelter him for life; I wish now that I had known how normal this is. One evening, having been desperate for some time alone, I was dressing on the riverbank after a swim when a couple in their late thirties meandered past at a pace surely only childless people keep. 'Been in yet?' the man asked, his long sandy hair escaping beneath a thick woollen hat. We exchanged a few words and they pottered on. I felt a pang of envy; that could have been me and Philip, taking an early evening stroll for no particular reason, hand in hand with no cares other than for each other. And then a wave of guilt; it was me who pushed for a child, me who wanted this. But when I got home I was greeted by the sweetest human being in the world, and the regrets and guilt melted away.

The third challenge is the gulf between fantasy and reality – how our expectations of ourselves, our births, our babies, our partners, and indeed of motherhood itself, the whole shebang – can be so vastly different to how we expected. I never expected to cry quite so much. Nor did I expect Philip to go through his own equally difficult *patrescence*, to coin a word. I didn't expect the physical symptoms, and I didn't expect to feel as incompetent, naive and lost as I did. This was one of the things that made me want to write this book; the conspiracy of silence that surrounds the postpartum period sets too many of us up for a fall. By talking more openly about it, we can start to bridge the gap between expectation and reality and, I hope, spend more time enjoying our tiny charges.

Lastly, Sacks describes the feelings of guilt and shame that we entertain, and our unwillingness to give up on perfection and, instead, accept being a 'good enough mother'. Like Imogen on page 325, a lot of us strive for perfection, or to be the ideal mother, whatever that may be – and it's impossible to achieve. The phrase 'the good enough mother' was coined by the British psychoanalyst and paediatrician Donald Winnicott, and should actually encourage us to embrace our failures, rather than feel like we're settling for something short of excellence. After observing thousands of mothers and babies, Donald decided that children actually benefit from their mothers failing them in manageable ways. Only when babies experience frustration and breaks in the empathy and attunement that they have with their mother do they develop a sense of the external world and how it will not always conform to their wishes. So, the next time you find your child crying in its cot when you've been out in the garden completely unaware, try not to feel guilty or blame yourself – Donald's theory gives you permission to consider it a lesson, instead.

Anna, who was among the first of her friends to have children, chose to go back to work at three months:
'Having had a baby, I remember thinking that everyone should do it at 21 when their life is still made up of flexible entities, because if you put it off until your life is full, you have so much more to give up. With your first baby, you also have no feeling for what you're aiming at, or the way developments happen in stages, each of which is finite. We don't live in mixed-age communities anymore. I'd never even seen or held a baby less than six months old – I was completely unaware. And the boredom was relentless. It's not the lack

of sleep, it's that your day turns into one long constant with no change in heart rate or contrast. It's just the same, for 24 hours. I'm not a jealous person, but I definitely was jealous of my husband going to work every day. The journey was so steep, and so slow and lonely in the first months, that I found myself working out my route 'back' to work (and 'normal' life). But I felt like I was a passenger to circumstance, nothing was in my control, even though I'd built up so many skills, ambitions and interests and developed so many aspects of my life. And then, suddenly, it shifted to feeling that maybe nothing really mattered apart from this, the baby. And then I thought, shit – maybe I am just supposed to be a brilliant mum and home-maker? I used to think working mums were more impressive people; now I know that there is no such duality, and that whichever you choose is completely valid. It's a huge hourly, daily, constant challenge, being a mum; my admiration for people has doubled and trebled every day.

'We talk about getting back but you don't ever get back – it's a whole new norm, with something completely different that you're working towards (or around, because it's a lot less linear with a child). "She's back at work already," people said about me when my baby was three months old and I went back part-time. It's the same as childbirth, with or without an epidural – there's this strange fascination with women's choices. One of the biggest problems is that men will never ever understand it – and how could they? The journey that women take, and the understanding and the responsibility that comes with it, is so huge – it's far longer and more winding than the journey the man takes. They still get to the same point, but while men get there more directly, women take every hairpin bend and then the very long slalom which

embeds a profound experience of the journey within their very being.

I didn't understand it before it happened to me. I still don't have many of the answers, I just know more of the challenges. Fifty per cent of our population will never understand any of this and, of the fifty per cent that do, only a few will question it. It's so weird that you can't escape your gender; it makes all of the narrative about equal pay and 'equality' feel completely ridiculous – we talk about things being the same but it can't be the same. From the moment we have children, we are different, and that should inform the choices we make up to that point. But if I had the choice of being the one who went through childbirth or not, it's such a powerful and monumental thing, I would choose to do it.'

(Re)defining yourself?

I like running for the same reasons I like writing; it requires no special equipment or preparation, can commence immediately, and you never know where it's going to take you. I think the reason I found it so hard not being able to run was that I no longer had a choice in the matter. It's not like I went running every day before I had a baby and suddenly it was taken from me. I would run whenever I felt like running, in the same way that I usually did whatever I wanted to in life; my experiences were governed by opportunities, not limitations. And then, overnight, this tiny, joyous creature shackled me to a wall.

Some of the constraints it imposed were good – in the long run, at least. Having a child means you have less time than you did previously and, as a result, you can either drop things that are important to you, or prune your lifestyle down to just the things that you value the most. Eventually, I did the latter and, since time is now so precious, almost everything I do – including relaxing and unwinding – has focus and intention.

My problem at the start, however, was that I was physically unable to do some of the things that I enjoyed the most. I'd read that I could run six to twelve weeks after the birth, but I could barely walk at that point without feeling like someone had taken the springs off my internal trampoline. I decided to leave it three months, then six months, then nine months. I began to think it would never be the same, so I turned to swimming instead.

In early spring, after an unseasonal bout of snow, I remember trotting down the steep bank to the river feeling giddy with trepidation. It was soggy and there was not a soul in sight as I dumped my towel in the mud, always in a rush to get in; the more time you have to think about getting into cold water, the harder it is. I gasped, breathing quickly; the water always surprises me and on this day in March it felt colder than it had in deep winter. When my breath returned to normal, I set off upstream. Large black-and-white cows grazed on the opposite bank as I swam against the current at a crawl. A minute or so later, I turned and floated downstream, then swam up again. I stayed in for no longer than a few minutes in total, but that shot of adrenaline and burst of effort helped me to feel like myself for days afterwards.

Looking back, I really don't understand the fixation I had with defining myself. It's not something I'd thought much about before, nor something I've given much thought to since – but it's something a lot of new mothers talk about. Nearly three years on, I'm still regularly shattered by the demands of parenting, work and marriage. I don't make the time to run or to swim as often as I'd like. And now another baby is on the way, and I'm about to go through it all again. I suppose I've adjusted; I'm myself no matter how I spend my time.

Becoming a parent can take away your self-assuredness and leave you feeling exposed – but it's temporary. As the barrage of dirty nappies slows and gives way to potties, beakers of cows' milk replace boobs, and broken nights become the exception rather than the rule, life takes on a form and shape that feels sustainable; the finish line that has been out of sight for so long suddenly appears on the horizon, and you develop a new assuredness and sense of joy. Like any challenge – think of Jasmin Paris's 268-mile non-stop winter mountain marathon – the more effort a thing requires, the greater the potential pay-off. Becoming a parent is no different in this regard: the challenge is befitting of the reward. If motherhood were easy, I'm not sure I'd like it so much.

Many women told me that it wasn't being a mum that they found most difficult, but not feeling like themselves. I know that feeling, but I also think that struggling with early motherhood can be a sign that you are being true to yourself. The woman I had become by the time I turned 35 did not, and will never, delight in nappies, sleep deprivation, leaky boobs and laundry – but I do love my baby.

Next time around, I hope I'll remember this; that it's all temporary, nothing stays the same, and that total exasperation and even desperation is, at times, perfectly normal and fine. The person you once thought of as yourself – with a career, ambitions, interests and an engaging social life – is still there, she's just taking a back seat for a short while.

24

Doing It Again

I finished writing this book just two weeks before my second baby was due. Exploring the most traumatic of the issues raised in the book with a growing baby inside me was, at times, unnerving. But, ultimately, the knowledge I gained from my research left me feeling stronger, and in a position to take positive action.

As I was putting the final words to paper, my oestrogen-saturated brain turned, inevitably, to labour, and how the body I had inhabited since my first birth would change again this time around. I yearned for the pregnancy to be over – for the pain in my hips and my right buttock to subside, for my belly to stop expanding ever outwards, and for the pressure on my bladder and bowel to ease. But a new ache was there in the background as well – the desire to meet, and to start to know, my child. I didn't feel that ache the last time around because I'd had no sense of what birth meant or what it would lead to. The second time, I could anticipate the intensity of the journey ahead of us and, despite my anatomical complaints, I was ready to face it.

I didn't feel as strong, in the literal sense, as I had before I first went into labour; each time your body goes through this, it comes out a little stretched and more prone to injury. 'I feel as pregnant now with weeks to go as I did ten days overdue last time!' I lamented to a physiotherapist friend.

'It's perfectly physiological and normal. It'll be annoying and less comfortable, but your body is just obeying the laws of nature,' she replied.

I will never again feel as invincible as I did before being pregnant; I'll never be able to leap around on a trampoline or run a marathon without thinking about my core strength first. But, mentally, I feel more stable, and better prepared.

Was it likely to be the same again, I wondered? Would I have another giant baby, that I'd have to push out with brute force? Or would I lie back in water and – aaaaaaah – breathe it out? Was it likely to be late, as my first was late? Would my pelvic floor suffer similarly again? And would my mind be more likely to stay on the right side of the raw and often indistinct line between equilibrium and depression in the weeks and months afterwards, if I avoided depression before? With excitement (and a degree of trepidation), I ferreted out answers to these questions and more.

What to expect from subsequent births

Gynaecologists and obstetricians agree that we are likely to experience physical symptoms earlier on in subsequent pregnancies, and that our bodies might then take longer to recover afterwards. But what about the labour – could it be quicker? Happily, yes. For first-timers, it usually takes eight to twelve hours to go from being more than three centimetres dilated to being fully dilated. For second- and third-timers, it typically takes half that; around five hours. Your body retains a memory of what it needs to do; your muscles already know what they had to learn on the job during the first labour.

Research shows that second babies are more likely than

first babies to be born on their due date. They are, on average, born slightly earlier – but only by 16 hours. Research suggests that babies conceived within a year of their brother or sister are likely to spend less time in the womb. And it does appear that once you've had one longer pregnancy, you're more likely to have another (which came as a relief – my first was ten days late, so I could feel relaxed about my deadline for this book).

When it comes to your perineum, you're less likely to tear if you've already given birth. A 2013 study found that your chance of emerging with your perineum intact is just less than 10 per cent the first time around, but a little over 30 per cent on your second, third or more birth. Just over 6 per cent of first-timers end up with a third- or fourth-degree tear in the UK, according to a 2014 study, compared with less than 2 per cent of women who've already had a vaginal birth (although many women opt for a caesarean after a serious tear, which may skew the figures – and if you did have a third- or fourth-degree tear the first time around, your risk of it recurring remains about the same as it was the first time, 6 per cent).

When it comes to pelvic floor damage, there's more good news; it's usually the first birth that does the deep structural damage, according to a 2014 study, so whilst you'll likely find that your pelvic floor is weaker due to stretching, any damage to the deep musculature is likely to have already occurred. If you've already learned about the pelvic floor muscles and how to train them, you'll be in a good position to rehabilitate them through exercise.

In less-good news for me, after our beast of a first-born, your second and third babies are statistically likely to be bigger than the first. Although it's not understood why, a second baby with the same father is likely to be about five ounces heavier than the first.

Birth spacing

Around the world, traditional cultures encourage pregnancy spacing of around two and a half or three years, which is in line with what modern scientific literature now endorses. The World Health Organization recommends a gap of 18 to 24 months between birth and conception, but a recent Canadian study suggests that 12 to 18 months is actually an ideal gap for most women. According to the WHO data, women who conceive again before 18 months have a slightly higher risk of having babies with reduced growth, preterm births and other physical and mental developmental issues – although these problems are statistically extremely rare now in developed countries, so don't let a shorter gap cause undue alarm.

Our understanding of why outcomes appear to be worse with a very short gap between pregnancies is limited, but it's thought that nutrient depletion, cervical incompetence (when the cervix is not strong enough to support the uterus and dilates prematurely), and the fact that scar tissue may not have fully healed are believed to play a role.

Of course, for some people, waiting 24 or even 18 months feels like a luxury they can't – or don't want to – afford. For others, choice doesn't factor; you just find yourself pregnant. If either of these scenarios applies to you, doctors and dieticians urge you to ensure your diet is rich in nutrients (see Chapter 9) and take a good prenatal multivitamin as a safety net. Physiotherapists encourage women to do as much as they can to support the strength in their core and pelvic floor whilst pregnant, to support their recovery after the second birth.

If you've experienced a miscarriage, there is even less of a need to worry about leaving a gap before trying again. In fact, a 2017 review found that a gap of less than six months carried a lower risk of miscarriage or preterm birth than an interval of six months or more. An interval of less than three months after pregnancy loss was associated with the lowest risk of subsequent miscarriage, leading experts to advise that you try again when it feels right to do so, rather than worry about leaving it a certain length of time.

Do we forget the pain of childbirth?

It's important that humans remember pain: it warns us of the things that can threaten and injure us, and the memory of pain and the resultant fear acts as a device to keep us alive. When it comes to childbirth, however, women the world over say that it's a pain that they forget; 'the amnesia of childbirth', as a perplexed new father once said to me.

It's very difficult to measure and compare pain because it's subjective but, on the whole, research suggests that many women start to recall the pain as less acute over time. This mirrors the feeling – known as the halo effect – that women have minutes after the birth, when their happiness quickly skews their experience of labour, and the joy of holding their newborn washes away all of those hours of weeping, groaning and pushing. Not all women get this, however. Those who've had a difficult birth and whose babies are rushed off for ventilation, for example, are never able to bask in the afterglow of labour. For these women, research suggests the pain, as they recall it, does not lessen over time. For women who had a negative experience of childbirth, the pain sometimes never diminishes in their minds.

Interestingly, according to one study, women who have epidurals report experiencing higher levels of pain than those who give birth without pain relief; pain is subjective, and it seems that women administered epidurals recall the moments of peak pain – before the anaesthetic kicked in (rather than averaging the pain out across the whole experience, a process that diminishes it).

Childbirth is like a marathon or any endurance trial in this regard; if it goes well, you tend to minimise the suffering you experienced. If it goes badly, or you are suddenly forced out of the race, you're more likely to focus on the worst points. Experiences that give great joy and achievement often involve equivalent amounts of hardship and struggle; in spite of the challenges, we still seek them out again. I've seen it in my job as a foreign correspondent, where journalists – my husband included – would put themselves in terrifying and hellish situations. (He once said he could 'never do this again' after a particularly harrowing experience during the Libyan civil war, but just a year later he was in Aleppo, facing far worse, covering the Syrian conflict.)

For me, there is nothing as difficult, and nothing as commensurately satisfying, as growing a baby, giving birth to it, and raising it – yet it's the most commonplace undertaking in the world. Maybe it's because of our tendency to seek out hardship, and then gloss over the worst of it once we're through it, that we largely fail to convey to our sisters, friends and daughters just how challenging early motherhood can be; the conspiracy of silence means that very few of us emerge from early motherhood feeling like we entered it prepared and well informed.

Doing it again after a traumatic birth

No matter what your first experience of birth was like, the feelings and emotions you now associate with pregnancy, labour and parenting from your first child may well arise in you again. If you had a traumatic birth, approaching labour can be extremely daunting – and can even put couples off having a second child. Occasionally, according to the Birth Trauma Association, the symptoms of PTSD from your first birth might not even occur until you start contemplating pregnancy again.

The Make Birth Better network, a collaboration of parents and professionals working to raise awareness around birth trauma, share women's birth stories on their Instagram page. Often, these stories are powerfully redemptive, as women overcome traumatic first births by having the labour they'd always wanted with their second. Of course, it doesn't always work out this way, but for many women the second birth ends up being therapeutic, superseding their experience of the first. This is why some midwives urge women to save the detailed birth plan for their second birth, which is likely to be more predictable.

If your last birth was traumatic, the Birth Trauma Association urges you to discuss it in a professional environment – either at a debrief from the hospital (something everyone is entitled to), or with a midwife, counsellor, health visitor or support group – before embarking on another pregnancy. You need to identify any symptoms that arise in you, like flashbacks, anger, guilt, anxiety or depression, and consider counselling or therapy with a specialist who can help you to come to terms with your experience and develop the resources you need for another pregnancy. Ensure you are supported by healthcare providers who you trust, and who are sensitive and respectful. You must feel safe and secure, and know that you have a right to be heard when you express your concerns. Take heart from the fact that experts say you're unlikely to have two traumatic birth experiences.

Mental health

If you had postnatal depression the first time around, you're more likely to experience it again; according to the Association for Post-Natal Illness (APNI), there's around a 50 per cent chance of recurrence after a subsequent birth, and this can make the decision to have another child a really difficult and complex one. However, there is also evidence that psychological support reduces the chances of recurrence. Two drug treatments are also available: injections and pessaries to support your levels of progesterone, and anti-depressants. Some doctors believe the use of anti-depressants in late pregnancy could be dangerous for the baby, while others believe the benefits outweigh the risks.

APNI advises that women who've had postnatal depression after a previous birth prepare for the fact that they're likely to have it again – warn friends and family, and establish a strong support network around you. If you do this, you'll be more likely to spot symptoms and seek treatment quickly, with a solid support base to help you through; and even if you're fine this time around, you won't have lost anything by being prepared.

A lot of women who have the most severe form of mental illness, postpartum psychosis – which affects around one in a thousand (see page 145) – go on to have more children, but there is about a 50 per cent risk that the condition will recur. But not having any more babies doesn't guarantee they'll stay well either, according to the Royal College of Psychiatrists; over half of women who had postpartum psychosis will go on to have another episode that isn't related to childbirth.

Self-care

As the countdown to my second birth ticked by, the agonising pain in my hips started keeping me up at night and I was limping, thanks to a sore gluteus (buttock) muscle. But, having researched this book, my physical health mattered more to me as I approached labour than almost anything else, so I did something I would never have done before and booked a private appointment with a chiropractor to see what they could do.

The decision to prioritise myself was not an easy one, but it was driven by the many women in this book who have urged me, and other new mothers, to put themselves first, and seek help before their physical or mental problems start getting them down. Having been through it once, I also knew what my body would soon have to endure, and what I would lose – albeit, I hoped, temporarily – in terms of physical fitness. I reminded myself that this was not the sort of race you want to start injured, if you can possibly avoid it.

Within a week of my first appointment with the chiropractor, I was walking without pain and only feeling stiffness at night, allowing me to enjoy our precious last few weeks as a family of three. It made a tremendous difference to how I felt at virtually all times of the day – I literally felt lighter.

There is no getting around the fact that private healthcare like this is expensive, and out of reach for a lot of people. But think back to that mind-boggling figure of £10,000, the average amount couples in the UK spend on their babies in the first year of life. Often the impact of making do with less of what doesn't matter (new stuff, extravagant food or expensive entertainment) in order to pay for healthcare can be far less costly to you, in terms of what does matter, than living with discomfort or injury. Prioritise yourself, and borrow what you can, shop at car boot sales if you need to, dress your baby in cast-offs, sing to them, and let them play with spoons.

Ultimately, we all want to give our children the best start in life, and one of the simplest ways to do that is to ensure that we, their mothers and fathers, are in good shape ourselves. I've started early, and plan to stick to it this time around.

Part 4

PREPARING YOUR PARTNER
TO SUPPORT YOU

In 2013 Robbie Williams told Graham Norton on his chat show that seeing his wife give birth 'was like my favourite pub burning down.' The audience laughed hard, while his wife fumed. It's a good gag – Robbie wasn't the first to use it – but it spares no thought for the pub's landlord who's lost everything and faces the arduous task of reconstructing it. The process of getting a baby out of a woman's body can, it's true, torpedo our most intimate, sensitive and secret but vital parts. 'Imagine your penis was torn in half in order to bring our baby into the world, and then you had to walk around with it like that for a month,' one friend said to her husband, who wanted to understand how she felt after the birth of their second child. It's not always easy for men to comprehend this.

Having a baby can be one of the most wonderful and exciting times for a couple, but it can also be challenging, particularly with the new responsibilities that lie ahead. Be aware of your partner's feelings, because becoming a parent represents a huge life change for them, too. And try to communicate clearly what you need. We as mums generally feel poorly prepared for this time ourselves, so how can we expect our partners to know how to help? If they have no real concept of the physical, mental and emotional changes we're dealing with, how can we expect them to empathise? I thought Philip and I would be fine – we'd navigated unpredictable urban warfare together in Central Africa, after all. But it turns out that Congolese guerrilla fighters don't have anything on a newborn baby when it comes to putting stress on a couple.

The issues that can crop up range from the surprising and entertaining to the deep-rooted, unpleasant, embarrassing and taboo – which is why we're not always great at talking about them, or tackling them. The women I've interviewed have almost unanimously spoken about how they didn't prioritise their own health in the early days, weeks and months of motherhood. Some struggled to find the words to describe how they were feeling, others were too embarrassed, and others still didn't recognise what was going on until it was too late.

In recent decades, society has put men in the front seat when it comes to a woman's labour and recovery from childbirth, and the care of new babies. This gives them many happy and intimate experiences that they would have been denied just a few decades ago – but our partners can also find early parenthood difficult, and society does not always prepare them well for their new role. Traditional family units are not there anymore; many mothers don't talk to their daughters about this stuff, let alone to their sons. Women reach for Google at the first sign of a problem rather than talking to a partner, friend or family member. And, when the adrenaline fades and we're mind-crushingly tired, we as mothers are not best placed to process what we're experiencing and communicate our needs.

Same-sex partners might find it easier to relate to each other in these circumstances, but life can still throw barriers in the way – for example, if one partner is going to work every day and the other has given up her career, or one carries the burden of physical transformation and the other remains unchanged.

The following, and final, chapter of this book is designed to bridge the gap between how we're often feeling and behaving as new mums and what our partners experience, so they can understand and support us better, rather than resent our behaviour. And it includes advice for partners on their own mental health – because, even if they love you, they won't be a great help if they're busy fighting demons themselves. If your partner wants to help you, they should read it, because if they have this knowledge, you might just be able to avoid some of the difficult and painful steps couples go through in understanding each other after a new baby arrives. Think of it as preemptive therapy that will help him or her to temper their reactions to you during this tricky period. As Gloria Anzaldúa, the Mexican-American feminist thinker wrote, 'The possibilities are numerous once we decide to act and not react.'

25

Advice for Partners

Childbirth is intense whatever the means of delivery; there's no getting around that. What we don't talk about is the fact that it doesn't end there. Preparations tend to lead up to the big push, and then skip ahead to the minutiae of child-rearing – but it's the long days, weeks, months, sometimes years that follow that can be the hardest for a woman; a time she may need to rebuild herself, literally and metaphorically, inside and out, whilst caring for a newborn, often alone. This time is known as the postnatal (or postpartum) period, and it refers to the six weeks, three months, six months, nine months, or even a year or more of a woman's life after her baby is born; there is no strict definition, and many health professionals say, *once postnatal, always postnatal.* For many women, it denotes the most intense and transformative journey she will ever take. Remember this if you get praised for taking two weeks off work or changing a nappy, or if the baby is crying at 4 a.m. and you feel resentful because you have to go to work that day. For many people, it feels infinitely harder to be at home with a newborn baby than it does to go to work.

The postnatal period is not just tricky for a woman; it can be one of the most difficult times in a couple's life. But, if you can try to understand what your partner is going through, temporarily set aside your ego, be endlessly kind, and help her to get what she needs, you'll be well-positioned to survive it. As London acupuncturist Ross J. Barr, who treats a lot of couples (including A-listers and royalty) believes, 'The mother is the key. If she's well-rested, nourished, calm and happy, everyone is. But if she's not in good condition, everyone is fucked.'

The first three chapters of this book describe the astonishing physical and mental feats that becoming a mother involves; read them and you'll feel even more awestruck by your partner and what she has achieved. The majority of it is written for women, to help them understand what they're going through and what they need. And this last section, based on dozens of interviews with fathers, mothers and health professionals, is written for new fathers and co-mothers, because societal changes mean they no longer stand aside while women handle the labour, recovery and childrearing.

It's important to remember that we as new mums often don't understand what's going on with our minds and bodies ourselves, so how are we to put these things into words? The sorts of things we face can be embarrassing, complicated, traumatic, personal and emotional. Our medical system typically doesn't prepare us for them, and nor do our friends and family; the physical and mental challenges and changes catch us off-guard as much as they do you, so we're not always in a great position to explain them. And even if we do seek help from our health system, our symptoms are too often brushed off as either inevitable consequences of childbirth, or things that just take time to resolve, which can leave us feeling foolish or demanding.

Whatever your situation, you'll probably find some of your partner's behaviour during the early weeks and months to be strange, saddening, concerning or just out of character. This section explains some of the things that might help you understand the drivers. You can then use the information to see why your partner might be reacting differently to you – not wanting any physical contact, crying more than usual, or being angry and anxious, for example – and to temper your reactions. It also suggests a number of practical things that you can do to make this time easier for her. I'm not saying all men like solving things but, let's be honest, many do.

Kindness is the best guiding principle. If you can always be kind – and it won't be easy when your partner's shouting at you for something you haven't done, or weeping because of something you have – things will be immeasurably easier. Ross J. Barr advises his male clients to 'suck it up' – the sleep deprivation, harsh words, emotional rollercoaster or absence of sex (or physical contact) – because if it's hard for you, it's harder for her. And it won't last; just swallow your pride for the time being. The gentler and more accepting you can be now, he says, the more content and less resentful your partner will be later on.

The aftermath

As said, women themselves don't usually have any idea what to expect after the birth. And if *we* don't have any idea of what to expect – the haemorrhoids, bleeding or leaky nipples, insomnia, mood swings, vaginal cuts and tears, infections, incontinence and bowel problems – then how on earth should you? We read and talk at length about the big push, when you finally get to meet your child, and then skip ahead to the details: what sort of baby monitor to get, whether or not to swaddle, what kind of baby wipes to buy. We spend hundreds (if not thousands) of pounds and weeks' worth of time preparing for the baby, but fail to realise that it's our bodies and minds that may require the most attention.

On top of the physical symptoms, some of us experience mental ones: a loss of identity and independence; a sense of claustrophobia and the ambivalence of feeling unable to leave your child but wanting nothing more than to be away from them; crashing hormones that result in the most monumental of come-downs; structural changes in our brains that put us on a new, baby-focused wavelength. The mental and physical upheaval is so colossal and ubiquitous that it raises really valid questions as to how and why no one really tries to prepare us for it the first time around.

Ancient Chinese medicine dictates that the best way to stop a baby crying is to treat the mother. Many new mothers – running on adrenaline and trying to be superheroes – need to be reminded of this.

Matt Coyne, author of Dummy, *a bestselling book on fatherhood:*
'I used to think that the theory that the Moon landing was a hoax was total bollocks, just because it required a huge amount of people to share a secret. I now think it's a distinct possibility given the conspiracy of silence about how horrendous labour is.'

After the birth, your partner will have a large internal wound on the inside of her uterus, where the placenta was previously attached. She'll be bleeding heavily, and her bodily functions (milk, wee and poo) will become a focal point. She may have a catheter, might struggle to go to the loo, or might leak. Personally, I couldn't hold a fart. Sitting down, or doing anything at all, will be excruciatingly painful. New mothers need the option of doing nothing but focusing on sleeping, resting and feeding their babies – for the first few weeks, at least.

If your partner is in hospital, you'd have thought she'd be well looked after and that you could relax and ready the home for her return. Sadly, it's not always so. Hospital maternity care can leave women feeling very lonely, sometimes without their babies anywhere near them, stuck with bad food and without the kindness, care and attention they need.

Many maternity care providers in the UK are very dedicated and try extremely hard to deliver good care – but they are underfunded and understaffed, and things do go wrong. Over a period of five years, the NHS recently paid out over £5 billion to compensate new mothers for what happened to them when things went wrong during childbirth. And postnatal care, which falls under the maternity care bracket, is particularly lacking; it's known as the 'Cinderella service' for the pitiful amount of funding it receives.

In France, every new mother understands the importance of rehabilitating her pelvic floor – the muscle that's responsible for controlling wee and poo, holding the organs of your pelvis in place, and sexual function – which can stretch by up to four times its length during birth. Every French woman, whether she had a caesarean or a vaginal birth, gets a course of one-on-one physiotherapy sessions beginning around six weeks after the birth, to ensure she recovers full control over her bladder and bowel and is left with no pain or dysfunction down there. The NHS offers no such thing (unless you have a severe birth injury); instead, too many women struggle on, concealing their symptoms – or trying to ignore them – for years until they get too problematic to hide or ignore.

A lot of the women I interviewed felt like discarded crisp packets after the birth, so intense and narrow was the medical establishment's focus on their baby. Listen to your partner, remember that her health matters as much as your baby's; be her best advocate and don't be afraid to ask questions of her healthcare team or demand better care so that she feels safe and looked after. If necessary, encourage her to ask questions of herself; her symptoms should be treated rather than accepted as a 'normal' side-effect of childbirth.

Her mental health

If the birth was difficult or she felt out of control or afraid during it, you may find she's more angry or irritable than usual. Birth is traumatic for roughly a third of all women, and anger and irritability are common by-products of this; it's often mild (but occasionally full-blown) PTSD. If there is ever a time to let her rant and rage, snipe and gripe, or snivel and weep, it's now. Try not to take it personally, and if it gets worse, or she doesn't level out within a couple of weeks, encourage her to talk to her midwife, GP or a counsellor or psychotherapist, some of whom accept self-referrals on the NHS.

In some cases, you can tell immediately after the birth that something isn't right – if she is delusional, for example, or had an extremely traumatic birth and isn't sleeping because of nightmares or anxiety. If this is the case, follow your instincts and contact your midwife or GP immediately; you can also go straight to A&E, where she should be seen by a psychiatric team. If a medical professional dismisses her and she gets worse, you must go back again. Severe postnatal depression and postpartum psychosis (see Chapter 10) can ebb and flow, and both are medical emergencies.

At the other end of the spectrum are the emotional ups and downs that affect almost all of us. 'Hormonal' is often construed as a condescending, catch-all term for weepy women. The cute phrase 'the baby blues' likewise belittles the physiological reality: after we give birth, the chemical balance in our brains changes almost overnight to such an extent that it triggers psychosis (in one in 1,000 mums), depression (in one in ten), anxiety (one in five) and temporary mood disorders (four in five). And it's the mildest of these, mood disorders, that we refer to as the baby blues.

Trust your instinct as to whether her mood swings, melancholy or irritability become something more entrenched and problematic, like severe anxiety or depression. And read Chapter 10 on postnatal mental health if you're worried and want to find out more. The field of postnatal mental health can be very hard to navigate; even euphoria, another recognised condition that may be linked to bipolar disorder, can be a problem as it leads to severe sleep deprivation, and it can culminate in a major crash.

Sleep can actually stave off some of these disorders; it improves your ability to cope with pretty much anything, and regularly getting less than seven hours a night (something most new parents consider a victory) has severe side-effects – it's as bad for your body as heavy drinking. Getting good sleep will often seem like a lost cause, but there are ways to help each other sleep more (see page 373). There's no shame in sleeping in different beds (or even on the sofa) or wearing ear plugs. You can even buy headphones designed for sleeping in. Take both of your shut-eye seriously, even from the outset when you're not feeling too bad, because sleep deprivation is cumulative.

> *Gareth, a father of two children, likens a new mother's emotional turmoil to a bereavement:*
> 'Their hormones will be all over the place, they'll be tired, they'll be hungry, they'll feel impotent with the baby, guilty and responsible – all these things that mums go through. It's almost like a bereavement in many ways, so you have to prepare yourself for a bit of emotional turmoil. If you're ready for it and you know it's coming, you might be able to temper your reactions.'

A word on ... crying

Your partner may cry rather a lot in the first few days, weeks and months. If she is still finding joy in things that would usually bring her pleasure – a sunny day, gurgling baby, juicy peach, or an unbroken night of sleep – then her crying is likely to be quite normal. If it seems that she can't climb out of her place of sadness and despair, then it might indicate anxiety or depression. Crying can even be a positive thing; a way of accepting difficult emotions and letting them out. I myself cry with relief. Almost every argument between me and my husband Philip ends with me in tears as I release the emotions that built up inside as we were fighting. It's taken him years to get used to this, and even now I still see that look of exasperation cross his face when, just as we've navigated our way out of a fight, I burst into tears. There are infinite ways in which a newborn baby can make a woman cry; try not to feel responsible, and try to quash the urge to fight it.

> *Clinical psychologist Dr Genevieve von Lob says many of us grew up in families where crying was seen as a weakness. We didn't have the kind of role models who*

could have normalised crying, and shown us how
cathartic tears can be:

'When women have just had a baby, they need space to shed
their own tears, without having to feel like they are responsible for managing their partner's feelings as well. Some men
may struggle to know how to respond, perhaps feeling an urge
to problem-solve or come up with solutions, when all a mother
really wants is to be given some comfort, or even space to
sit with her messy feelings. I've worked with many men who
had difficulty connecting with their own tears because they'd
learned growing up that boys shouldn't cry. The key thing is
for new mothers and fathers to learn to listen to each other
and communicate the kind of support they need from each
other as clearly and kindly as possible.'

Physical healing

The best thing my partner ever did for me in the days after
the birth was tell me to stop being prudish, lie down and
spread my legs. I was worried about how I was healing down
there but trying to put on a brave face. He suggested he take
a look. I resisted and tried to change the subject, but he was
calm, gentle and adamant: 'Come on, let's examine you.' Mol-
lified, I lay back. And, afterwards, I felt immeasurably better.
When I later told a pelvic health physio about this gesture of
support, her eyes widened in surprise. 'And he's not a doctor?
That's amazing. I must remember to tell my sons to do that
when they become fathers,' she said.

I appreciate that this might not be for everyone, but it is
practical to help your partner to know how she's recovering
(if she had a vaginal delivery), and there can be an intimacy
to the gesture that breaks down awkwardness, and shows

your partner that her recovery is something you are willing to share.

If you're not the stop-being-prudish-and-spread-your-legs type, or your partner would be uncomfortable with it, talking about how she's feeling – and simply listening – can be a huge help. The healing process is different for everyone, and new mums often keep their fears and problems to themselves. A gentle sense of humour can make it easier; one couple I know privately called her undercarriage 'frankengina' after two particularly difficult births.

Some people worry that by discussing these things they'll lose some magic or sexual intrigue. The reality is, however, that this is no time for squeamishness. These aren't problems that disappear overnight – a majority of women find sex painful after childbirth, and 30 per cent are still finding it uncomfortable at six months; the stats on incontinence issues are similar – and if you can't talk about them, you may find that they put some distance between you. On the contrary, if you do talk about any issues she has, you'll probably find it brings you closer and improves your sex life in the long run. As experts have told me, if it's done right, being completely open about what's happened or how she's healing, gives you an opportunity to have greater awareness and understanding – and, as a result of that, more empathy.

What to expect after a vaginal birth

As maternity budgets are cut across the country, your partner might find that you're the only person who offers to take a look at how she's healing. In the past, midwives visited new mums pretty much every day for a month. Now, after a typical labour, a midwife might see a woman at home once or twice, then in a clinic, before discharging her after a week or so, and it may be that they don't offer to examine her at all.

If you do take a look at your partner after a vaginal birth, expect the vulva, the area around her vagina, to look swollen, open – like it's yawning, as one physio advised – and more 'frilly' than before. The perineum between the back of the vagina and the bum might be less defined because of stretching. And you may be able to see the ridges of the vagina that are usually hidden inside. The anus is likely to be engorged (it might stay that way for a while), and she might have a haemorrhoid or two. You might also see a tear and stitches. It is extraordinary how quickly it can heal, however. While it does, just help her look out for any sign of infection: increasing pain, a bad smell, hot and inflamed tissue or feeling generally unwell with a temperature are all indicators of a problem.

Going to the loo can be painful, as can pretty much anything, from walking to sitting down. You can help her take regular baths to soothe the area and keep it clean; water can be very healing, and adding salt or essential oils like lavender and tea tree oil may promote healing and lift the spirits. The pelvic floor, the muscles that support all of our pelvic organs, are usually stretched and weak after birth; this might mean she has problems with incontinence (urine, wind or stools). Try to make her feel comfortable talking to you about these issues; gynaecologists I spoke with estimated that up to two-thirds of women keep incontinence issues secret. But there is no need for her to live with it long term if the problem doesn't go away by itself. Remember that many women don't realise that these are common problems. This is uncharted territory for a lot of us, so we may need reminding that, beyond 12 weeks, any ongoing symptoms, although common, are *not* a normal state of affairs, and we shouldn't accept them. Physiotherapy can usually cure physical symptoms as well as prevent problems later in life; if she's the reticent type, getting her to open up about this stuff now could help her access treatment and save her from worse problems down the line.

What to expect after a caesarean

If your partner had a caesarean, you'll have heard the advice – she isn't to lift anything heavy, climb stairs, or do anything much for several weeks. This means that the heavy lifting – both literally and metaphorically – will fall on you. She may feel back to normal after just a few weeks, but doing too much too soon can hamper her progress. Recovery usually takes at least six weeks – and a lot of women still feel tenderness in their scar tissue, the pelvis or during sex for months or more afterwards. Even though her vagina was saved the trauma of stretching to accommodate a baby, her insides are still reconfiguring themselves after months of pregnancy, and problems with bladder control, haemorrhoids and pain during sex are still common – the baby came out of the opposite end of the same tube, after all.

Emergency caesareans also leave women more susceptible to depression and birth trauma, or can make them feel like they somehow failed. You can help by encouraging her to talk about what happened, and by reading up on mental health problems (see page 124) so that you're prepared if her mood swings do become something more entrenched.

Pelvic floor primer

I had no idea what the pelvic floor was before becoming pregnant – and I'm not unusual in that. It's often not until we have babies that we become aware of this invisible body part, a hammock of muscle that's strung between our legs, front to back, from pubic bone to coccyx. In men and women, it holds the sex and digestive organs in place, allows you to control your wee and poo, and improves your orgasms. It's essential, in short. And pregnancy and childbirth can subject it to a fairly major traction injury.

Pelvic floor problems affect almost all women who've been pregnant (and many who haven't) at some point in their lives. Common symptoms include prolapses (when one of your pelvic organs – the bladder, womb or bowel – drops down with gravity because it's not getting enough support), bladder or bowel incontinence, constipation, laxity and pain in the pelvis or hypersensitivity around the vagina.

To repeat, these problems are common but not normal and your partner shouldn't go without treatment in the long term. Not only can physical symptoms affect a woman's self-esteem, relationship, sex drive and ability to enjoy herself, but they can also turn into far more serious problems in the future.

Nutrition and recovery

If your partner is breastfeeding, this will be the most nutritionally demanding time in her life. What she eats, and her physical and mental recovery, are closely linked. Iron deficiency is particularly common and can cause fatigue and increase the risk of postnatal depression. There are also a host of proteins, vitamins and minerals that are essential for tissue healing. When you're keeping the fridge and freezer stocked, think about this. The basic rule endorsed by nutritionists is to focus on nutrient-rich food. That means carbs like bread, pasta, rice and cereal shouldn't be the mainstay of her diet. She needs some carbs for energy – on top of breast-feeding and recovery, there are the demands of looking after a newborn – but she really needs the nutrients that come from eating a variety of fruit, vegetables (especially leafy greens), nuts, seeds, meat (organ meats like liver make the ultimate post-natal meal – and may be more palatable than the placenta!), soya-bean products like tofu, dairy, fish, shellfish (which is particularly rich in iron) and pulses. Nutritionists recommend you encourage your partner to take a supplement as a back-up; the symptoms of nutritional deficiencies can be the same as the symptoms for postnatal depression – or just sheer exhaustion – so they often get missed.

A word on ... postnatal depletion

The Australian doctor, Oscar Serrallach, noticed something was wrong with his wife after she had their third child. Her confidence, energy, brain function and digestive health were all in very bad shape, but he didn't know why. He realised that her condition was far from rare – many of his female patients over the years had shown the same constellation of symptoms – so he turned to the medical discipline for answers, but found none. After years of research, he coined the phrase postnatal depletion. Oscar believes the nutritional and energy demands on a woman during pregnancy and beyond can sap her of her life force and have both physical and mental long-term consequences. A woman needs to recover physically after having a child; if she doesn't do this, she might find she's running on empty for years afterwards. In his book, *The Postnatal Depletion Cure*, he advocates a multi-pronged solution including better sleep, mindful exercise like yoga, and emotional support, but the core pillar of it is nutrition (and good-quality supplements), which should be within everyone's grasp – particularly as the NHS gives free multivitamins to women receiving benefits with children under one. He also advocates getting as much help as you can: 'You can't have too much support (and a babysitter is a lot cheaper than a divorce),' as he once told Gwyneth Paltrow's website, goop.

Sex

Your body has not changed, but hers has been through a life-changing physiological and psychological transformation – she's come full circle, from sex, through nine months of pregnancy, to its ultimate, awesome and most intimate result. Your journey back to where you started, with a sex life, might take a little time; while most women are technically OK to have sex again after six weeks, many find this too soon. Our bodies need time to heal and recalibrate. Sometimes it's exhaustion and time constraints, other times it's physical injuries. Whatever the root cause, you can help your partner to get the support she needs and get things back on track.

Sex is about more than physical pleasure – it also brings intimacy. You may want to find alternative ways to hold on to that intimacy for the sake of your relationship, whilst her body (and mind) recover. Give her a foot massage, or take a bath or shower together. Heck, one couple I know used to sit on the sofa and hold hands while she got over her third-degree tear; the recovery process can require great kindness and patience. Sex therapists recommend 'outercourse', which can be anything from massage and just kissing, to fingering and oral sex. Find what your partner's comfortable with and meet her there.

Accepting that her body feels new and different, and then discovering it together, can provide an opportunity for intimacy; but your partner may need some reassurance that you're in it with her and that you won't be freaked out by any changes. If you feel comfortable doing so, offer to massage any scar tissue or areas where she feels pain. And if you're having sex and something hurts or malfunctions, talk about it; if she's happy to, you can try another angle or position; physiotherapists talk candidly about the need to 'steer in a slightly different direction'.

Her physical symptoms, coupled with exhaustion and the rigours of breastfeeding, may, however, mean that your touch is the last thing she wants. If this is the message you're getting – if she flinches at your hand and wants to crawl into bed, alone, at 8 p.m. every night – try not to feel rejected. It's very common, particularly if a woman is breastfeeding, for her to feel 'touched out'. As a new mum, it can feel like your body is no longer your own; not content with destroying a woman's overall strength and physical integrity, her miniature marauder then lays claim to individual body parts, kneading, nibbling, scratching and sucking them with abandon. I found this new physical intimacy with my baby so arresting and all-consuming that the last thing I wanted was someone else having a go at my boobs.

If it's intimacy that you're missing, demonstrate that you don't expect it to develop into sex but just want to hold her. It might help to remind yourself that your adult life together is not over, it'll just be different for a while. And if you communicate well about things like this, none of these challenges should be too much. It's also possible that you have little or no sex drive for a while; studies show that fatigue, stress, and lack of time are the top three reasons for partners – whether male or female – to go off sex for a while. Rather than worry about it, experts recommend you focus first on getting both of you back into good physical and mental condition.

Access to healthcare

While women are getting better at asking for what we want and need, the postpartum period can be something of a twilight zone, where we forget everything we know about looking after ourselves and exist in a world outside of logic. Many of us prioritise our child at the expense of our own recovery, even though recovering is the most important thing we can do for that child.

At around six weeks after the birth, all women in the UK should see their GP (or sometimes nurse) for a check-up on their physical and mental health. At its best, this appointment presents an important opportunity for the medical system to pick up on any problems – physical, mental or emotional – that a woman may be experiencing, and to refer her where necessary for specialist care, or monitor her to prevent the problems from escalating. At its worst, however, it is 'a complete waste of time', as some women and even GPs say – a box-ticking exercise that skims over problems and doesn't provide the time for either clinician or patient to explore any of their issues satisfactorily. Chapter 14 presents expert advice on how to get the most out of this appointment. You can also help your partner to make the best of it by talking to her about her concerns in advance, so she feels prepared and ready to discuss them. Encourage her to have a checklist of issues she'd like to address and questions she wants to ask during the appointment.

If, after your partner's six-week check, something still doesn't feel right to her – if she still has any pain, discomfort or concerns about her healing that the NHS isn't addressing – help her to investigate where she can get support. In the NHS system, that may mean not taking no for an answer, and encouraging her to go back to the GP again and again until she gets the support she needs. Alternatively, if you have the means to pay for it, there are brilliant women's health physiotherapists, counsellors and psychotherapists specialising in postnatal health all over the country; they're just not always available on the NHS. Invest in your partner's reproductive health in the same way you would anything else.

In terms of her recovery, women's health physios (also known as pelvic health physios) recommend that, if something doesn't feel right three months after the birth, it's unlikely to resolve on its own and she should seek support. If it's a physical problem, physiotherapy is usually a good place to start – and many physios offer free telephone consultations to work out what help you need.

My husband recently confessed that he still doesn't know how to help me when I talk about the problems I've had with my pelvic floor – it's not like he can massage it. I never told him that a good physiotherapist could have fixed it straight after the birth. Or that I didn't want to ask him, in those early months when everything felt so difficult, to take time off work to look after the baby so that I could spend money we didn't have on private healthcare. I fell into the universal trap of putting my baby's health (and my partner's) before my own – and by doing so didn't help anyone in the long run.

Boobs, breastmilk and bottles

> *Marcus Berkmann, author of* Fatherhood: The Truth*:*
> *'Some fathers, I have to say, don't like it. Having formed an intimate alliance with the mother's breasts, they see their place taken by this greedy little latecomer who appears to have instant access to the precious globes.'*

If your partner decides to breastfeed, you should know that, although it can be one of the most beautiful and intimate experiences a woman will ever have, it is not always easy. We wrongly assume that breastfeeding a suckling infant is a serene activity. Often, it is not. Words that may more accurately describe it, in the early days at least, are messy, painful, awkward and difficult.

Breastfeeding is a common source of anxiety for new mums. Personally, I found it most upsetting when my baby wouldn't feed from me; being rejected by your own child whilst you sit there with one boob hanging out is a uniquely ignominious defeat. And I felt ashamed by the way I seemed to leak milk everywhere and constantly stank of the stale stuff. No one warns you that milk can start gushing out at inopportune moments; whenever you hear a baby cry, or when you orgasm, for example. For this reason, breastfeeding women wear breast pads that contain the leakage; think sanitary towels, but for boobs. Accidents still, however, happen – usually when you're wearing a light grey top – and you're left with two humiliating dark circles that broadcast the purpose and position of your nipples.

It's very common to experience pain at the start when breastfeeding; this tends to go away after a few weeks. Sore or even cracked and bleeding nipples are very common while you get the hang of it, and the advice is usually to feed through the pain to prevent the milk drying up. Be sensitive to all of this and don't expect to be fondling her breasts anytime soon.

If your partner is having problems, you can also watch to see where she may be going wrong. You'll quickly discover that it's all about *the latch* – the attachment your baby's mouth forms with the nipple. The word 'suckling' doesn't do this process justice: rather than use its lips to suck, the baby needs to take a deep gulp of breast, particularly lower breast, with its mouth wide open, to feed correctly. Look at the La Leche League website – they're like the Samaritans for breastfeeding mothers – or read the breastfeeding advice given to you by your midwife or health visitor, and see if you can spot where things are going wrong. Because you have a different angle on them, you're in a good place to help. During the early weeks, for example, Philip would often watch and tell me when our son couldn't tilt his head back to feed, because he could see more clearly than I could, my view being mostly obscured by gigantic boobs. Sometimes, it can be as simple as the fact that the baby can't tip his head back adequately, that their gullet is twisted, or that they're not taking a big-enough gulp of the lower boob. It's an art, and may take some practice. If you see that she's getting stressed with feeding and think it would help, you could offer to take the baby while she recalibrates.

Given the amount of time the average mother spends feeding her child, it can be a source of postural problems that can cause back, neck or shoulder pain. You can help by making sure she has enough cushions and a supportive chair. You can also make her aware of her posture if you notice that she's all twisted up. Experts recommend that, rather than bend down to the baby, you lift it up on cushions so that it's at the right height to drink. When sitting to feed, the mother's back should be supported, her hips higher than her knees and, ideally, both feet should be flat on the floor.

Breastfeeding women also get tremendously thirsty, and often find they can't get to a bottle or tap whilst feeding. Offer her water and herbal teas wherever you can – in a bottle or cup with a lid, if necessary, to avoid spillages. In Part 3 of this book, I described how the poet Hollie McNish's partner would dot water bottles all over the house after their baby arrived, so that no matter where Hollie got stuck during the long nights of feeding, she'd find a spill-proof source of hydration within arm's reach.

If your baby – or babies – are bottle fed, it goes without saying that you can also get up in the night to share the night feeds. (The positive side of this, however, as the journalist Marcus Berkmann points out in his book, *Fatherhood: The Truth*, is that you might get access to your partner's breasts rather sooner than if she were breastfeeding.) If your baby is breastfed and you want it to drink from a bottle as well as a boob, however, you as the father or co-mother are often the best person to introduce it; the mother is too closely associated with boobs. Once your partner's boobs are producing milk in line with the baby's needs, usually after about four weeks, she can try expressing milk and you can try feeding the baby with a bottle. Experts recommend that you keep it up, at least once a week or so, to ensure the baby doesn't forget how to feed from a bottle.

When our little boy was five weeks old, we spent a

night at a foreign correspondents' club in London whilst I received an award for a story I'd recently published. Philip had spent days getting the baby used to bottle feeding, and I expressed milk for the weekend while Philip fed it to the baby. He fed him in the toilets, in our small room, the corridors, and even squatting on the pavement (where, at one point, a man entering the club mistook him for a beggar and offered him a pound). It was exhausting and stressful for us both, but also a small but important triumph and, for me, a chink of freedom. After that, we blithely assumed our baby drank milk from a bottle. But, by the time we tried it again (when he was almost four months old), he wasn't having any of it. Despite repeated attempts by Philip to get him back on the bottle over a number of months, that weekend in West London is the only time he's ever drunk from a bottle – and it will remain so for the rest of his life.

If you and your partner want the freedom of handing your baby over to relatives or a carer before they are at least six months old and can drink from a cup, don't make the same mistake as us. And if you want the option of being able to take over at night when your partner is at the end of her tether with sleep deprivation, you'll need your baby to drink from a bottle. Bottle feeding doesn't matter to everyone, but to me – and to my mum, who was desperate to help more but couldn't feed the baby – it did. And we fluffed it.

Bottle feeding is not always easy to start with, either. Babies can be remarkably bad at the one thing they're supposed to know how to do: drink milk. They might gulp air, then start crying because they have wind in their bellies, which they're unable to expel. But they're also still hungry, so they keep trying to feed, which only makes the wind situation worse. If this happens, keep calm, and burp them. Then try again. It'll get easier with time; before you know it, they'll be holding their own bottle while you and your partner read the newspaper.

Burping

Even babies that don't gulp take in small quantities of air when they feed. As these small quantities build up, the air can become painful in their little tummies, and they need your help to get it out. This usually happens after a feed, but sometimes you need to stop halfway and burp the baby in order to finish the feed.

I have male friends who consider themselves baby-gas aficionados, such is the pride they take in having mastered the infant burp. Everyone develops their own technique, but favourites include sitting the baby on your knee, holding them upright and drawing little circles with their upper body, putting them face-down over your knees and patting or rubbing their back, or jigging around or walking up and down the stairs as you hold their upper body but let their legs hang free. You can also lie them on their fronts, which often allows them to burp themselves.

You have to keep burping your baby until they can do it themselves, which is anywhere between four and nine months. It's tedious and time-consuming but essential work, because a baby with bad wind can be a very noisy baby indeed.

Sleep

Sleep is the panacea of parenting; get a good night, and everything feels OK. One more bad night, and you're on the edge of reason. When sleep was bad and both Philip and I were equally sleep-deprived, it was a recipe for disaster. I recall one evening when all three of us were in tears at the same time. We had a spare room but he always insisted on sleeping in the same bed as me. 'The walls are too thin, I'll hear it anyway,' he protested. Or, sometimes, 'I don't want to be that couple.' We are now living in a new house with walls made from stone rather than plasterboard and, as we hurtle towards baby number two, we've got over *not wanting to be that couple* and will gratefully enjoy separate beds sometimes when the new baby arrives. I'm also gunning for a white-noise machine that pumps out soothing static – not for the baby, but to allow at least one of us to sleep through even the shrillest of cries. Or wax earplugs. If you take sleep seriously, you'll be more likely to take a strategic approach to it, so that there's never a time when both of you reach peak exhaustion. Respect sleep's healing powers, and remember how sleep deprivation can twist your interpretations.

As Ross J. Barr has seen, both in himself and in his clients, there may be times in the day when you both feel wrecked, and are each under different pressures. 'When people are that tired, they become very much about themselves; their rationale, their perception of what's going on in the whole household, becomes what's going on with them. Try to notice when one of you is more fucked than the other, and that's when you need to be at your kindest. That can be carried throughout all of those early months and years; it really makes a difference and prevents resentment from building up.'

Harry puts the working partner's role into perspective:
'Try to acknowledge that you might feel knackered, you've been at work all day, and you're the breadwinner, but in

actual fact you've got it easy; it's hard being at home all day with a newborn baby – it's easier to go to work. So temper the frustration that you feel when you're tired and you're up at three in the morning again and you think, "I've got to be up in three hours to go to work and you haven't, you can have a lie in." It's not like that.'

Sleep tips

Everyone handles sleep deprivation differently. Try to find whatever works best for you as a couple, whether it's sleeping in separate rooms so that at least one of you is well rested, or – if you're bottle feeding – taking it in turns to get up with the baby.

- If you can split the night shifts, do; even with breastfed babies, partners can do the last feed of the day, giving the baby expressed milk or formula around 10 p.m., while the mum gets an early night. Split it like that and she could get six hours of sleep in before having to feed again at 2 a.m. Meanwhile you put earplugs in or listen to white noise if you're a light sleeper, and sleep for the rest of the night.
- Beware the witching hour; for some reason, arguments often seem to start in the evening after the baby has gone to bed, and there is nothing more annoying than an argument you can't wrap up when you're both desperate to get to sleep yourselves. If you are tempted to bring up something even remotely sensitive, don't do it in the hour or two before you go to bed. The last thing you want is to miss out on sleep because you're still stewing on something.

- If your partner is the one getting up in the night to feed the baby, you could offer to get up in the morning whenever possible (after she's fed them, if she's breastfeeding) and give her another hour or so in bed. Or try to give her time to nap – or at least rest – after lunch at the weekends. Depending on your partner's personality, she may take some persuading, but if she doesn't make up for the lost sleep, she'll start to find everything harder – which may mean you will too.

- If you have other children, you can be the one to get up with them in the mornings, or stay up after your partner goes to bed to do whatever needs doing around the house.

The shitty end of things

The partner's role in the business of babies is not well-defined at the very start. Newborn babies are usually pretty simple, after all – they eat, vomit, sleep and poo. 'I fed Jess, she fed the baby,' is how my husband describes our first weeks postpartum. We ate sumptuously, and I did little in the way of clearing up. This is a pretty common division of labour, because someone still needs to cook and clean, and the mum is resting and feeding the baby. Nappies, too, need to be changed; there is no earthly reason why partners should not change nappies, particularly at the start. I remember a trades-man saying to my husband, 'Do you change nappies, mate? Argh, I couldn't.' He meant it kindly enough, but it left me seething; did he think his wife enjoyed the mustard-yellow crap? And then there's the laundry. Such a lot of laundry. So there really is a lot that you can do during the early phase.

The trouble is, it's all at the shitty end of things – dirty sheets, nappies, bums and dishes. Within weeks of the birth, Philip's face had received our son's wee, poo and vomit; he'd even spent one morning cleaning a generous layer of crap off the inside of our radiator with a toothbrush. While you're out on a limb cleaning up and doing housework, it can feel like the mother and baby are doing all the bonding (in other words, lazing around) whilst doing the hallowed work of feeding. And rightly so, it's fair to argue – the woman has grown this baby, gone through childbirth, and is now nourishing it with her own body. But, as a number of people have said to me, it's also important that we give men a role as a father in the early weeks and months. 'The perception of men is not always considered, and that can manifest in anxiety in pregnancy, through the birth, to the postnatal period, when they may feel rejected and left out,' says Grace Thomas, who leads midwifery education at Cardiff University.

At the start, you can hold the baby, take it out for walks in a sling or pushchair, change and bathe it, and feed it (if you can) from a bottle. If it's just breastfed, you'll find the gaps in between its feeds quickly get longer, so you'll be able to go further without worrying it'll get hungry. A lot of couples find their newborns get more demanding after the first few weeks, which is when a lot of partners go back to work. If and when you do go back to work, remember how lonely it can be at home with a newborn. I've spoken to women who would yearn for their partner to walk through the door at the end of the day and take the baby out of their hands, such was their need for a break. Other women piled pressure on themselves to get the baby ready for bed by the time their partner came home. You may need to be ultra-sensitive and a bit of a detective to work out what your partner needs as she might not be explicit about it. We tend to try to manage everything – the cooking, housework, laundry, social life and admin – on top of the baby, and to feel guilty if we let something drop.

Psychologists recognise that it's not always easy for fathers to carve out their role when the mother–baby relationship is at its most intense; back in 1999, academics coined the phrase 'maternal gatekeeping' for the way mothers inhibit fathers' involvement in their children's lives. Often, and particularly in the early days, the mother only allows the father to contribute in a very specific or minor way and, in doing so, they can set a negative precedent for the future. Impotent is a word I've heard a lot of partners use to describe how they felt when it came to their newborn; unable to help. But then you also hear, further down the line, a lot of mums bemoaning the fact that their partners do nothing. This may not sound like much of a problem to you – my husband jokes that he was delighted to be hamstrung by his absence of boobs – but not splitting the tasks more evenly in the early weeks and months sets a precedent that can lead to your partner resenting you. We have a very long way to go before men and women reach anything like an equal footing in terms of parenting; of all the men entitled to take shared parental leave in 2017–8, just over 1 per cent took it. That's not an easy statistic for women – particularly those who've given up their careers – to swallow.

Redress the imbalance wherever you can. Like mums, dads need this time to bond with their baby and to learn to care for and comfort them. If you don't get that time, you'll either find you don't have the confidence to help further down the line, or that you are just a bit inept because you haven't had any practice. We all know couples where the woman handles pretty much everything and the man just goes to work, and where that woman quietly resents him for it. If you can find a way to handle more than just the crap, seize it – for the long-term good of your relationships, with your partner and your child.

'It's amazing how many useless men there are,' as Ross J. Barr said. 'Establishing the kindness principle sets an early precedent so that you start to do more anyway, whether it be feeding your child, bathing your child, or taking them out for walks. You'll build your confidence, feel better about yourself as a man, and feel like you're taking care of your family in a way that's not just the "financial provider" bracket. Also, if you know your wife respects you and doesn't resent you, it makes a big difference, doesn't it?!'

Giving her a break

'It is as difficult to leave your children as it is to stay with them.'

Rachel Cusk, *A Life's Work*

Ambivalence is something you get used to as a new parent; the contradictory feelings you have for your offspring that dictate you want never, ever to leave them, but also want to be rid of them, sometimes for good. Often, the greatest gift you can give a new mum is to insist that you take the baby for a walk or a nap in its pushchair while she has a bath, sleeps, works, reads, even paints her nails – whatever she wants to do, as long as it's her time, and it's undisturbed.

Paradoxically, you may encounter some resistance to your efforts to help. After birth, there are some women who calmly nap while the baby naps and graciously accept every offer of help, but a lot of us run on adrenaline; we become superheroes, functioning on four hours of sleep a night and going running whilst the baby naps. But the adrenaline doesn't last and, at some point, we may crash. If your partner fits into the latter category, you might need to ask a few times if you want to give her a break. Alternatively, phrase it to say you'd *like* to do something with the baby on your own, rather than offer to help and have your offer declined.

The other thing to know is that the meaning of 'a break' can change quite drastically when you become a mother. I remember Philip being so diligent about making me supper that I started to resent the time he spent cooking. A month in, I would have done anything for a child-free hour in the kitchen, or even an hour on my own to clean the house. One exasperated friend found herself dropping hints for her husband to learn some twenty-minute recipes: 'But they fell on deaf ears as he used every pot and pan in the kitchen over the course of an hour. And after the meal he'd disappear to clean up.' In those early months, I used to jump at the chance to go to the supermarket alone, just for the novelty of being out, without a baby. It's easy to fall into roles – one of you works, one doesn't; one does the cooking, one feeds the baby – but it's also easy to start resenting your partner for their role. As said before, try to share the jobs and mix it up where you can.

Loss of freedom and identity

Desmond Morris, a British zoologist, once designed a simple experiment to ascertain whether women and men react differently to babies. If a human being sees something they like, their pupils generally dilate; if they see something they dislike, the pupils contract. Desmond found that a woman's pupils, whether or not she has had children, dilate when she sees a picture of a baby. In men, it is only those who've had children whose eyes dilate. The pupils of a man who hasn't had children (whether he's single or not) 'show a strong *negative* response, their pupils shrinking as if to shut out the picture of the baby before them', as Desmond wrote in his 1991 book, *Babywatching*.

To gloss over the fact that men can go through their own crisis of identity when they become fathers would be disingenuous. You might feel stressed at the new burdens your child has placed on you (particularly when they seem to give so little back), you may find yourself mourning your freedom, or just feel fed up with your partner being miserable, exhausted or anxious, or just talking about the baby all the time. On the whole, the challenges are greater for your partner, however. She has likely lost so much more than her evenings and weekends; the list of things that a woman may feel she's given up (albeit temporarily) includes her physical integrity, mental stability, self-identity and career. *She* may not like talking about the baby all the time any more than you do. And the more proficient a woman is in life, the harder she can find it to suddenly be shackled to a baby. Often, women are at their most creative when they start having children, or have finally reached a point where they know who they are and what they want from their careers. And then – bang – it's gone, everything is put on hold, while the average partner is praised for spending two weeks at home before going back to work.

Your mental health

There are clear physiological reasons why we need to look out for a woman's mental health around the time she gives birth – but the father or co-parent's mental health is also important, not least because they need to be in a good place to support her. Becoming a parent is a big transition for both partners and can lead to depression and other problems in men, so take care of yourself. And if your partner had a difficult birth, don't belittle your own experience and its impact on you.

Trauma

Anyone present in the room during birth can experience trauma; rates are particularly high amongst midwives. Trauma was identified as far back as Ancient Greece, but came into sharper focus during the First World War, when some 80,000 men were treated for shell shock. Our understanding of trauma – now known as post-traumatic stress disorder, or PTSD – has changed dramatically since then, but a hundred years on we still face one major problem: getting people – men, in particular – to recognise it. A lot of men still see it as soft, or namby-pamby, to admit they're struggling and need help. And the problem is no different when it comes to childbirth.

Birth doesn't have to be medically problematic to leave you or your partner feeling disturbed. The most straightforward birth in the world can leave someone feeling traumatised because they felt out of control. Afterwards, their feelings are too often dismissed as insignificant, when what they really need is validation.

No one knows how many men are affected by birth trauma but there is a growing body of evidence to show that men can find childbirth extremely distressing. A 2017 article by two British clinical psychologists concluded that 'it is essential for maternity services to routinely attend to the needs of fathers in their own right before, during and after childbirth'. However, just like with our armed forces – and my journalist colleagues in conflict zones – 'masculinity ideology may act as a barrier to men accessing help', as the psychologists wrote. If you are struggling – if you feel numb with shock, or keep replaying events in your mind, experience flashbacks or nightmares, become anxious, angry or fearful, and have trouble sleeping – talk to someone you trust, or to your midwife or health visitor. Mental health is now a huge part of what midwives learn about, and increasingly that includes yours, as the father or co-mother.

Aled is a GP who'd spent part of his training on a labour ward – but rather than make his wife's first birth easier, his professional experience made it harder:
'It was a pretty typical hospital birth – she failed to progress and the baby's heart rate slowed down. They decided to monitor the heart rate so put a probe on the baby's scalp. As a doctor, I could tell it wasn't right but I didn't want to be that person who was really demanding. The sister was a bit panicky, and she tried to use a suction cup. It was traumatic because we knew he was in distress and it could have led to brain damage or death. After his birth, at about 2 a.m., they went to the ward and I came home. I walked into the ward in the morning, sat on the edge of the bed, and just broke down in tears; it was the release, I guess, that she and he were actually OK. I'd get flashbacks and, for a little while afterwards, I'd have moments of thinking, crikey, it could have been so much worse. Should I have been more pushy with the midwives, as opposed to being completely passive, I wondered? I always try to be passive in hospitals, but what if...? For some

weeks, I'd get recurring thoughts and moments of heightened anxiety, and then I'd remember – no, it's all fine. But if he'd not been fine, it would have haunted me.'

Depression in new fathers

Mark Williams, author and campaigner for fathers' mental health:
'A dad with postnatal depression comes across as a bad dad.'

Depression often goes undiagnosed in men. A conservative estimate of the number of new fathers it affects is 10 per cent, but a recent Swedish study suggested it was more like 22 per cent. Either way, between one in five and one in ten men get depressed after they become fathers. It's unclear as to exactly why. Some argue that it is the result of unaddressed issues that have built up over time; others believe it's more akin to postnatal depression in women, brought on by a combination of factors including hormonal changes. Just like a woman, a man's hormone levels change as he goes through life. In all mammals that share the burden of childcare, males experience a drop in testosterone levels around the birth of a child. The largest study of this phenomenon to date found that, not only do men with young children have less testosterone, but those who do the most childcare have the lowest levels – although that isn't meant as an advert for doing less childcare! Having lower levels of testosterone is linked to depression in men – and to lethargy and disinterest in general – while higher levels of testosterone are linked to stress. The cause and effect in fathers is not clear: it could be that lower testosterone levels are the cause of new fathers' depression, or that those with lower levels take on more childcare, and it's this that makes them more susceptible to it. Either way, it suggests that having a baby does put men at increased risk of some of the same depressive symptoms that new mums face, so keep an eye out for this.

There is, however, an understandable reluctance amongst the biggest healthcare providers and watchdogs to acknowledge postnatal depression in new fathers as 'postnatal depression'. The NICE guidelines for postnatal depression are explicitly for women, and the NHS refers to 'paternal depression' or the 'baby blues' instead. If you are struggling to enjoy the things you would normally enjoy, have trouble sleeping, lose your appetite or feel very tired, or if you are unduly sad, guilty, cranky, withdrawn or feeling isolated, you might be depressed – and it needs resolving. Read up on the subject, talk to your GP, a friend or family member, prioritise exercise, sleep and your diet, or book a private appointment with a counsellor or psychotherapist.

Sophie spent months worrying about her husband's mental health after their first baby:
'I remember the health visitor asking, how are you coping? Are you enjoying being a mum? I'm fine, I said, swallowing tears. To be honest I'm more worried about my husband, who is finding it really difficult. She just smiled at me – a look that said, I hear you, sister – and then moved on to her next task. I didn't bring it up again, but I'd desperately wanted her to ask more about him and his mental health. There was no way he was going to see anyone about it, so it felt like my job to try to help him. Telling the midwife that he was finding it difficult was my cry for help. I was struggling, but not because of the baby – because my husband wasn't himself. He was very down about his life in general, easily stressed, and

unable to cope when things went wrong. He told me a number of times that it felt like his life was over, and at least once he said he thought about suicide. My rock, the person who'd always been there to tell me things would work out and held my hand through challenges, had crumbled when I needed him the most. Sure, I was often difficult myself – anxious, illogical, utterly exhausted, or fed up – but which new mother isn't? I was looking after a newborn baby; that's what they do to you. I needed him to step back and see that it wouldn't be like this forever; to hold me tight and say it will be OK; to indulge my tears then make us a cup of tea or take the baby out for a walk. Instead, he would become sad, stressed, angry or defensive. As a result, most of my mental energy went into worrying about him. Luckily, we had a straightforward baby, otherwise I don't know how we'd have coped.'

If your partner has postnatal mental health problems

If your partner has postnatal depression, anxiety or psychosis (see Chapter 10), it's likely to affect you, too. It's only recently, however, that people have started to recognise this – and that it can start a chain reaction that eventually breaks up families. It's obviously vital that she gets help, but you may need help too.

In late 2018, the NHS announced a new policy: if a new mum has postnatal depression, anxiety or psychosis, her partner will be given a mental health check and offered support should they need it. The NHS described this as 'radical action', and the Fatherhood Institute, which lobbies for fathers' rights, welcomed it, noting that it was 'the first time the NHS has formally acknowledged fathers' powerful impact on mother and infant'. But, they added, health systems have yet to include partners formally in maternity care. We still need fairer policies for mums and dads.

> *Rhian Hall, creator of the website You, Me and PND, describes the power of simply saying 'OK' or 'I understand' to your partner, when they open up about their darkest thoughts and fears:*
> 'Listeners don't need to validate or add anything in response. Simply listening in non-judgement, and perhaps giving a hug, will provide huge relief. Just the fact that the listener hasn't gasped or shown revulsion is very powerful. These thoughts have likely bored holes in the thinker's mind. The listener's response has shown them that "thoughts are just thoughts". They no longer seem so formidable.'

Afterword

I went into labour with my second child on my due date, two weeks to the day after I finished writing this book. Whilst I'd experienced issues after my first birth, the labour itself was uncomplicated – I would even stretch to use the word enjoyable. I thought this qualified me for a similarly uncomplicated second, which is, in part, why I chose to give birth at home. But it wasn't to be – and my experience serves as a poignant personal reminder of how unpredictable childbirth can be.

I felt the first contractions around 9 p.m. We called the midwife and expected her to come immediately but by 11.30 p.m. no one had arrived and I was already in transition, every contraction bringing me to the brink of despair with the pain and exhaustion.

When two midwives eventually arrived together, around midnight, they found the baby's vital signs were not as expected. 'I've got decells' – said one, her shorthand for a decelerating heartbeat. 'We need to get to hospital.'

Then she examined me. I was almost fully dilated; it was too late, the baby was coming now.

'Can I push? Should I push?' I asked.

'Yes,' they both said, as I prepared to draw heavily again on the gas and air they'd just set up in our bedroom.

A few minutes later, the baby was born. But there was no cry, no struggling limbs or blinking eyes. The little boy did not breathe.

In all the time I'd spent researching this book and focusing on the risks of labour to my own body, I had scarcely considered the risks for my baby: the fact that he or she might not survive; that they might not be healthy, or could suffer irreparable damage during the birth. Everything I'd been writing, about prioritising a mother's health and wellbeing, was suddenly cast into irrelevance. I was ready to endure anything myself if only it could save him right now.

For months, I'd been interviewing women and writing about the psychological aspects of birth trauma without having experienced it myself. And now I was living it, watching myself watch panicked midwives trying to resuscitate a tiny grey body on our bedroom floor.

I stayed on my hands and knees on the bed while Philip held me tightly around the shoulders, providing an anchor for my soaring grief. I listened to the terrible, unfamiliar sounds that I was making as if they were coming from somebody else.

'Come on, boy,' the midwives kept repeating under their breath, as they urged him to establish his breathing. 'Where is that ambulance?' We waited for ten excruciating minutes before it arrived.

At some point the placenta came out. 'It hurts,' I remember crying, knowing that it was the least of my problems, but feeling so saturated by pain that it was impossible to take on anymore.

The paramedics were calm and professional. The act of standing up and walking to the ambulance helped me to recover myself and I was soon in a hospital surrounded by a team of paediatricians. Then Philip and I were in a room on the labour ward, but without our baby. We couldn't see him until the laboratory opened the next day to process my coronavirus test. Meanwhile, our baby was in intensive care, where he remained for five days; one day's worth of interventions, and a further four days spent undoing them. The days were punctuated by the sounding of alarms from the many machines attached to him, which alerted us to unbearable realities – that he'd stopped breathing again, his oxygen levels were too low, or his heart rate had dropped too far. Weeks later, we learned that there was nothing in particular wrong with him – he just hadn't established breathing well at birth, likely due to my 'precipitous' – in other words, very fast – labour.

After all the tubes were removed and the sensors detached from our baby, the doctors were happy that our son was healthy, and the nurses were happy that he was feeding well. Seven days after leaving our home in an ambulance, I arrived home, now with a family of four. Philip had removed all traces of the birth from our bedroom – fresh flowers on the dresser, the bloody sheets scrubbed clean – but, sleeping there on that first night, I still felt just how close we had come to tragedy within these four stone walls.

Trauma is insidious. I hadn't noticed it at first – sleeping at the hospital in a single room on the ward, I felt oddly calm and strong. It was at home that the nightmares started. I dreamt of escaping an Islamic terrorist attack in a shopping centre with a new baby in my arms, a throwback to our life in Nairobi where Somali terror group Al Shabaab would conduct regular bomb and grenade attacks. The dreams I had interlaced many different aspects of my emotional life; how I can be too quick to blame myself, prioritise others and belittle my own difficult experiences. When I dreamed of taking our baby to hospital in an ambulance with his hand in a ziplock freezer bag, berating myself for letting it detach, I knew I needed to do something about it.

A brilliant psychotherapist took me through a trauma treatment called EMDR (see Chapter 10) and it was transformational; the results were immediate. In our session that dealt with the birth, I spent an hour sobbing without speaking as I recalled and explored all of the thoughts and feelings I'd experienced during, and following, the birth. Afterwards, I felt hollowed out by the emotion I'd expressed, but also lighter, because the emotional baggage – the trauma – attached to what had happened was gone.

Now, when I talk about what happened, the once-familiar well of tears and catch in my throat never comes. It's not that I feel detached from the memory – it is still a part of me, and of my family's collective experience – but it no longer looms over me, threatening to disturb my inner equilibrium and sense of control.

Our baby is alive and is healthy. I will forever be grateful for that. But I will also never underestimate how lucky I was to have access to exceptional neonatal healthcare, such a supportive family, and to be able to afford private mental-health support.

I've applied a lot of what I learned by writing this book to my second postpartum journey. It hasn't been without incident but, on the whole, it's been very smooth. Given that it was such a quick labour, my body was in surprisingly good shape afterwards. The predictions held true, that the damage had already been done; my first baby established the route, and my second merely had to navigate it. Indeed, he shot out 'like a rat out of a drainpipe', to borrow the phrase my father uses to describe my younger sister's birth. My pelvic floor didn't feel markedly different afterwards, compared with the 'inter-war' years; and my abdominal muscles hadn't left their post either. The biggest challenge this time has been helping our toddler adjust to the new arrival – which might have something to do with why the baby is so low maintenance; I wouldn't go so far as to say that he's ignored, but he's certainly very grateful of any attention he receives.

Despite my best efforts, however, I must confess that my six-week check-up with the doctor was, at best, perfunctory, and at worst, a joke. Even with all the promises I'd made myself to make the six-week check really count this time around (see Chapter 14), and my fervent request for an in-person appointment, it ended up being a phone call with a nurse that lasted all of six minutes. This was ostensibly, at least in part, due to coronavirus restrictions, although the British Medical Association had made it clear that mother and baby checks should not be impacted by the pandemic and should continue as usual. For the psychological impact of the birth, I was told to contact a local charity who mostly help women who've had stillbirths. This was not what I needed, which is why I sought private support. And, to rehabilitate my pelvic floor so that I could do impact sports like running again, I was referred to an incontinence clinic, even though I don't have any active incontinence anymore. Months later, I have yet to hear from them.

Were we to live in a wealthy borough of London, perhaps it would have been different. Perhaps not. Having researched and written this book, I have learned what to look for, what to ask for, and where to push in order to get the services that we all should be receiving. I can't help but think that if, armed with this knowledge, I am still unable to get that care, it bodes very badly for everyone else.

I can only conclude that there are some things we won't be able to change alone, which is why we need to work together to bring about systemic change; by being more open, and seeking treatment wherever necessary. The postnatal issues we're talking about – from trauma to pelvic floor problems – are afflictions and injuries like any other condition, and the health system should be resourced to treat them as such, rather than belittling and misunderstanding them.

What have I learned? Firstly, that we mustn't just sit on our problems (literally, or metaphorically). We need to share them in order to find solutions to them, and to act before things get worse in later life; remember that incontinence is one of the top reasons for admission to nursing homes in this country. Don't be afraid to question what you're told and challenge the status quo. Childbirth does leave scars, but don't associate those scars with weakness, fragility or shame. The body is strong, capable, adaptable and resilient (and, yes, there is a mnemonic for that – SCAR). Women's health is an exciting and burgeoning field of healthcare, but it needs to empower women to make their own choices about their bodies, not cow or shame them into doing, or not doing, a certain thing. As it stands, most of us don't even know about the need for the many women's health specialists until after we give birth, when we're suddenly granted entry to this secret club. Only after I gave birth to my first-born did my mum friends start talking about prolapses, incontinence issues, psychological trauma and postnatal depression. We need to be talking to women about these things before they give birth, so they're prepared for it, and in a position to access whatever help they need. And we need to vote for governments that will invest in healthcare, so that services aren't eroded by staffing and budgetary issues.

Secondly, postnatal recovery is about far more than just physical issues; it includes an enormous life adjustment that takes time to understand. Whatever you're feeling during this time is totally valid, and the chances are there will be someone, somewhere, going through the same thing.

Finally, all is far from lost. More and more midwives, therapists, doctors and nurses are choosing to focus on postnatal health. The specialist care that women need now exists (even if you might have to pay for it). But not all solutions involve expensive appointments; some of the best researchers and practitioners are sharing their expertise in books, at gyms and fitness studios, podcasts and online (see Resources). Use it! Brilliant academics such as John DeLancey are working to make childbirth safer, predicting outcomes so that women can make choices about how and where to give birth based on actual data. Many obstetricians, gynaecologists and midwives are working incredibly hard to keep making birth better, despite dwindling budgets. Physiotherapists are coming up with new, evidence-based approaches that aim to make anything possible, no matter what your injury. And the private sector is rising to meet the demand as well, with brands such as Elvie challenging tech companies to make products for women that empower, rather than disempower, them. Remember the 'Kegel renaissance' foretold by urologist Dr Andrew Siegel? This is it.

Beloved as they are, small children limit us quite enough without the physical and mental impediments their births can impose on our bodies and minds. Invest in your recovery and get back to doing what you love. Believe me, your child will thank you. Their health is paramount, but yours is pretty important to them, too.

Acknowledgements

This book is the product of hundreds of hours of unsparing and achingly honest interviews and conversations with women who have achieved the extraordinary feat of bringing new life into the world. I could not be more grateful to each of you for trusting me with your experiences of motherhood, childbirth and recovery. You are role models and sources of inspiration, helping to make our world a safer, happier, place. Thank you for your candour; it is both what we share and our counterpoints that I have found so interesting and inspiring. Speaking out, in particular about traumatic or painful experiences, requires bravery, and you have it in spades.

Countless professionals from all walks of postnatal health have contributed their wisdom and experience to these pages; dedicated obstetricians, midwives, GPs, psychotherapists, physiotherapists, doulas, nutritionists, acupuncturists and other experts. I am tremendously thankful to each of you – for your time, skill, and inspiring sense of purpose in improving women's health; it has been a long struggle, as Sandra said to me, but the current strides in progress are hard to ignore.

Professor Mike Keighley at MASIC, Dr John DeLancey, Clare Bourne, Ross J. Barr and the fabulous team of physiotherapists at Liverpool Women's Hospital, you are leading lights in the field of women's health and I am honoured that you believed in this book enough to give your time and energy so generously. Kate Walsh and Elizabeth Braga, you are beyond brilliant.

When I was eleven years old, my first ever English teacher, Mr Moule, asked me to send him a copy of my first book when I wrote it. Mr Moule, I haven't forgotten. And I may never have actually written a book without Alex Perry's guidance over the years. Alex, you were the first editor to invest time in me, and your passion, prose, humour and counsel have kept me going when it felt like I was getting nowhere. Tessa Laughton, your strategic vision gave me a huge boost just when I needed it and I hope we work together again soon.

After five years overseas, we moved in 2016 to the hills above Llangollen, in North Wales. To all of the wonderful people who've helped us to settle – and to build a family – in this valley and beyond, for the support you've extended, the care you've given to our children and the advice you've given along the way, thank you. And doubly so to those whose stories provided the original inspiration for this book. At times it felt like women's health was the only thing I had to talk about, but even then you kept inviting me over for cake, cups of tea, and the occasional gin.

Peter and Mary Greenwood, your collective expertise and wisdom has been invaluable, and becoming your neighbour was indeed serendipitous. Thank you for such diligent and intelligent reading. And for accepting that I start sentences with conjunctions.

During the difficult week that we spent with our second-born in intensive care following his birth, our friends and neighbours here went out of their way to deliver care packages and keep our toddler entertained. Thank you. Living in our small rural community, I was lucky to have the same midwife prenatally and postnatally for both babies (although sadly not for the actual births). I hope more women can one day have the sort of support we received from Mai.

My agent Ed Wilson at Johnson and Alcock was among the first to recognise the book's potential and has shepherded it through many iterations to become what it is today. Ed, you believed in me long before I was actually ready to write a book, and you believed unflinchingly in this particular project from its inception. Thank you for your acumen, steady hand and staying power, and for your unwavering support.

I can still feel the frisson of my first meeting with Rebecca Gray, my publisher, and Cindy Chan, my editor, at Profile Books, when we discussed how important, necessary, and helpful *After Birth* could be. You were the perfect people to receive the baton from Ed, and to help develop my proposal into what it is today. Thank you for your commitment to helping women everywhere. Cindy, your insights and instincts have always been pitch perfect. Despite everything I preach about women asserting themselves and their rights, I still felt a little trepidation when I told you I was pregnant. Cindy and Rebecca, you exemplify the equality we should all take for granted as women; you gave me your full confidence that

Acknowledgements

I would manage to juggle pregnancy and early motherhood with the book's writing and editing processes, and I am forever indebted to you for making sure I got enough of that precious, irreplaceable time with my newborn baby.

Helena Caldon, your meticulous eye and sense of rhythm transformed my manuscript into a book and stilled my last-minute anxieties; it was an absolute pleasure to work with you. Lottie Fyfe at Profile, you orchestrated everything so immaculately, one could almost be tricked into thinking that it was easy to produce a book. Anna-Marie Fitzgerald, your energy and capacity for ideas is exhilarating and I'm so glad that it's you getting these issues out there for women to read about. Thank you to Ali Nadal, Jonathan Harley, Ilona Jasiewicz, Sam Johnson and Ben Murphy. So much work goes on behind the scenes at Profile to make it all run smoothly, I am endlessly grateful to everyone there. Jo Goodberry, your illustrations are fabulous. And Anna Morrison, the cover is perfect.

This book was several years in the making, but I committed it to paper during the 2020 coronavirus pandemic, with nurseries closed and pregnant with our second child. I am extremely grateful to the Journalist's Charity for extending support to us when we needed it the most – what you do is incalculably valuable. The Author's Foundation, the charitable arm of the Society of Authors, is one of the only other organisations offering grants to writers for works in progress. It's thanks to an award from you that I could afford the time I needed at my desk – during a pandemic, with a tiny baby – to finish the book, so thank you.

None of this would have been possible without the people who looked after Finlay and, later, Hugo with such care while I was scribbling away – Roxy, the staff at Moreton, and Charlotte – and, of course, my husband, who gave so graciously of his time when I was on a deadline. Dearest Phil, this book is for you. I ask the indulgence of the women who read it for my dedicating it to a man – but you're an extraordinary man (who knows almost as much about women's health as I do by now) and my best friend. Phil – my deepest gratitude for your rock-solid love and support, your exquisite photographs that somehow encapsulate the essence of our lives, and your devotion to raising our boys, reading my first drafts, and tidying up my endless trail of tea mugs.

To my sister, Nerissa – at times, I imagined I was writing this for you. Thank you for all your love and encouragement. And to my parents, Mum and Dad, who have read almost as many of my first drafts as Phil. You are the kindest, most dedicated advocates I could hope for. You have always been, and will always be there for me – like little shoulder angels forever whispering in my ear, 'You can do it, Jess.'

Lastly, it was giving birth that set me on the journey of creating this book. To Finlay and Hugo, whose births book-end these pages: thank you for the ever-changing, ever-challenging, ever-glorious voyage of discovery. I love you.

Llandynan, February 2021

Bibliography

There are thousands of books about the first days, weeks and months of being a parent, but most focus on the baby, not on you. The books about postnatal healing – many of them excellent – have until now been quite niche, focusing on either nutrition (such as *The First Forty Days*) or naturopathic healing (*The Fourth Trimester*). Many of them have been invaluable in researching this book and are mentioned here. Unfortunately, I didn't read any of them when I had my first baby – I was clueless back then – so have only become something of an expert after the fact.

From Rachel Cusk's searingly honest and funny laments, to Jane Simpson's no-nonsense *Pelvic Floor Bible*, I urge you to look up whichever of these books appeals to you (apart from *The Best Friends' Guide to ... Pregnancy*, which I wouldn't recommend, but have included here because I quote it in the book).

Marcus Berkmann, *Fatherhood: The Truth*, Vermilion, 2005
Luce Brett, *PMSL: Or How I Literally Pissed Myself Laughing and Survived the Last Taboo to Tell the Tale*, Green Tree, 2020
Bill Bryson, *The Body: A Guide for Occupants*, Doubleday, 2019
Rachel Cusk, *A Life's Work: On Becoming a Mother*, Faber & Faber, 2008
Laura Dockrill, *What Have I Done?*, Square Peg, 2020
Anne Enright, *Making Babies: Stumbling into Motherhood*, Vintage, 2005
Eric Franklin, *Pelvic Power*, Princeton Book Company, 2003
Beccy Hands & Alexis Stickland, *The Little Book of Self-Care for New Mums*, Vermilion, 2018
Maisie Hill, *Period Power*, Green Tree, 2019
Milli Hill, *Give Birth Like a Feminist*, HQ, 2019
Vicki Iovine, *The Best Friends' Guide to ... Pregnancy*, Bloomsbury, 2011
Kimberly Ann Johnson, *The Fourth Trimester*, Shambhala, 2017

After Birth

Dr Genevieve von Lob, *Happy Parent, Happy Child*, Corgi, 2018

Hollie McNish, *Nobody Told Me*, Fleet, 2020

Lily Nichols, *Real Food for Pregnancy*, Lily Nichols, 2018

Heng Ou, *The First Forty Days*, Stewart, Tabori & Chang, 2016

Alexandra Sacks & Catherine Birndorf, *What No One Tells You*, Orion
    Spring, 2019

Oscar Serrallach, *The Postnatal Depletion Cure*, Sphere, 2018

Jane Simpson, *The Pelvic Floor Bible*, Penguin Life, 2019

Amy Stein, *Heal Pelvic Pain*, McGraw-Hill Education, 2008

Clover Stroud, *My Wild and Sleepless Nights*, Doubleday, 2020

Matthew Walker, *Why We Sleep*, Penguin, 2018

Zainab Yate, *When Breastfeeding Sucks: What you need to know about
    nursing aversion and agitation*, Pinter & Martin Ltd, 2020

Resources

There are a growing number of organisations dedicated to making childbirth and postpartum care better for women. They have been invaluable to me as a researcher, and also to the millions of others they have helped through no-nonsense advice, taboo-busting stories and tireless campaign work. There are also thousands of professional individuals across the world who are fighting for better care, and better access to care, often by making good information freely available through podcasts, apps, interactive websites, YouTube videos and social media channels. Some of these resources are listed below.

Action on Postpartum Psychosis (APP), the national charity supporting women and families of those affected by post-natal psychosis: www.app-network.org

Biamother, a holistic wellness app for new and expectant mums, made by women's health experts: https://biamother.com

Birthrights, a UK charity that works to ensure women receive the respect and dignity they deserve in pregnancy and childbirth: www.birthrights.org.uk/about-us/

The Body Mechanic Sarah Keates Andrews' exercise videos: www.youtube.com/channel/UC4faYeewKIQa6ah9E8o3qTA

Breastfeeding Aversion, a website run by Zainab Yate, a public health expert who experienced breastfeeding aversion herself: https://www.breastfeedingaversion.com

Breastfeeding Basics, a website run by a lactation consultant, provides comprehensive advice on issues such as oversupply: https://www.breastfeedingbasics.com/articles/oversupply-too-much-breast-milk

British Association for Counselling and Psychotherapy's therapist
  directory: www.bacp.co.uk/search/Therapists

Elvie the femtech brand's YouTube channel, which hosts expert advice
  as well as free prenatal and postnatal Pilates: www.youtube.com/
  channel/UCW0UFX2elO3DE09cdP4Y78Q

Fix Flat Feet, a website full of free resources to fix flat feet, set up by an
  American physiotherapist, James Speck: https://www.fixflatfeet.
  com

FODMAP diet advice: https://www.ibsdiets.org

The Great British Public Toilet Map: https://www.toiletmap.org.uk

The Laura Mitchell Method of Relaxation download from Pelvic,
  Obstetric and Gynaecological Physiotherapy: https://pogp.csp.org.
  uk/system/files/publication_files/POGP-Mitchell.pdf

Make Birth Better, a collective of experts on a mission to end birth
  trauma: www.makebirthbetter.org

MASIC Foundation, the UK charity for supporting women who
  suffered third- and fourth-degree tears, resulting in incontinence:
  https://masic.org.uk

Mind, UK mental health charity that provides advice and
  support on issues including perinatal mental health: www.
  mind.org.uk/information-support/types-of-mental-health-
  problems/postnatal-depression-and-perinatal-mental-health/
  about-maternal-mental-health-problems/

Motherhood Sessions podcast, hosted by psychiatrist Alexandra Sacks:
  https://gimletmedia.com/shows/motherhood-sessions/episodes

The Mummy MOT, company that offers a specialist postnatal
  examination for women following birth founded by physiotherapist
  Maria Elliot: www.themummymot.com

MUTU System, an NHS-endorsed online exercise programme for new
  mums: https://mutusystem.co.uk

My Confident Bladder, an interactive website designed by Janis Miller,
  Professor of Obstetrics and Gynaecology at the University of
  Michigan, that teaches skills and techniques to improve bladder
  control: www.myconfidentbladder.com

Pelvic floor training workout by Kari Bø, physical therapist and exercise
  scientist at the Norwegian School of Sports Sciences: www.youtube.
  com/watch?v=3Tt2XOjjUIQ

Pregnancy Related Pelvic Girdle Pain For mothers to be and new mothers, leaflet published by the Royal College of Obstetricians and Gynaecologists: https://pogp.csp.org.uk/publications/pregnancy-related-pelvic-girdle-pain-mothers-be-new-mothers

Royal College of Obstetricians and Gynaecologists patient advice pages, including patient information leaflets: www.rcog.org.uk/en/patients/

Squeezy, the NHS-endorsed app to support people with pelvic floor exercise programmes: www.squeezyapp.com

UK Council for Psychotherapy's find a therapist service: www.psychotherapy.org.uk/find-a-therapist/

The Women's Health Podcast, hosted by physiotherapist Antony Lo: https://womenshealthpodcast.info

You, Me and PND, a website created by Rhian Hall, featuring her animation about postnatal depression, Hope and the Black Balloon: www.youmeandpnd.com

Index

JHM indicates Jessica Hatcher-Moore.